Hiba Moussaoui

EPIDEMIOLOGY OF DIGESTIVE CANCERS IN ALGERIA

Hiba Moussaoui

EPIDEMIOLOGY OF DIGESTIVE CANCERS IN ALGERIA

EAST AND SOUTHEAST REGION 2014 - 2018

ScienciaScripts

Cover image: www.ingimage.com

This book is a translation from the original published under ISBN 978-620-3-43673-0.

Publisher:
Sciencia Scripts
is a trademark of
Dodo Books Indian Ocean Ltd. and OmniScriptum S.R.L publishing group

120 High Road, East Finchley, London, N2 9ED, United Kingdom
Str. Armeneasca 28/1, office 1, Chisinau MD-2012, Republic of Moldova, Europe
Printed at: see last page
ISBN: 978-620-5-72434-7

Contents

INTRODUCTION

The International Agency for Research on Cancer (IARC) estimates that one in five men and one in six women worldwide will develop cancer in their lifetime, and that one in eight men and one in eleven women will die from their disease.

The incidence of cancer is still high in developed countries due to a high incidence of tumours associated with smoking and lifestyle. However, in these countries, cancer mortality rates have begun to decline due to a decrease in smoking prevalence, improved early detection and advances in cancer treatment.

In Algeria, at a time when a notable decrease in infectious diseases is beginning to be recorded, thanks to the various national programmes set up over the last few decades, we are witnessing a real epidemiological transition marked by the beginning of the demographic transition, the increase in life expectancy, the transformation of the environment and changes in lifestyle. Cancer and other chronic non-communicable diseases are now a public health priority.

Current trends point to the need for strategies to counter the continued growth of this scourge. This strategy should be based on the "cancer plans", to give a new dynamic in the management of all aspects related to prevention, therapy and information. The "National Cancer Plan (NCP) 2015-2019" is the ideal tool to achieve this goal.
The main objective of this plan is to reduce cancer deaths by identifying risk factors and by early prevention (national screening programmes for the most important sites).
The secondary objectives are multiple, such as the development of the information system, palliative care, quality of life and equity in access to care.
For a good management of oncological pathology, it is necessary to have an adequate information system; the cancer register is the ideal tool.

The CNP (2015 - 2019) has institutionalized Population Cancer Registries in each wilaya and organized a national network articulated in three regions (west, centre and east with a network of national actors). [1]
Cancer registries provide a useful data bank for physicians and policy makers at local and national levels. Incidence data from each registry allows comparison between the different wilayas covered by a cancer registry.
This tool will allow the investigation of disparities in the geographical distribution of the main sites, and will prompt the conduct of epidemiological studies with an etiological focus. They will give reliable indications on the cancer profile via incidence rates, trends and survival[2] . The results of these studies are very important for decision making at the wilaya, regional and national levels. These data can be shared internationally and provide visibility to the country's health information efforts.
Globally, cancers are among the leading causes of morbidity and mortality. In 2012, the number of new cancer cases was 14.1 million and the number of cancer deaths was 8.2 million (3). The number of new cases is expected to increase by about 70% over the next 2 decades.
Cancer is the second leading cause of death in the world, claiming 8.8 million lives in 2015 (almost one in six deaths worldwide is due to cancer). About 70% of cancer deaths occur in low- and middle-income countries.
About one third of cancer deaths are due to the 5 main behavioural and dietary risk factors; high body mass index, low fruit and vegetable consumption, lack of physical exercise, smoking and

alcohol consumption[4] . Smoking is the most important risk factor for cancer accounting for about 22% of all cancer deaths[5] .

Digestive cancers are a major global public health problem, due to their frequency and severity. The responsibility of the environment in the development of certain cancers, such as those of the digestive system, is well established[6] . They represent 20% of the number of new cases of all cancers and 15% of cancer deaths in the world[7] ; their epidemiology is characterised by large geographical and demographic variations.

Colorectal cancer is the most common digestive cancer, with an estimated 1,400,000 new cases in 2015, representing about 15% of all cancers worldwide[8] . Mortality from stomach cancer remains high, although in recent years its incidence has been declining worldwide[9] . Hepatocellular carcinoma (HCC) is a malignancy with a rapidly increasing incidence and high mortality with extremely disappointing treatment[7] ; resophageal cancer is also a common cancer with high mortality worldwide, cancers of the pancreas, anal canal, gallbladder and small intestine are relatively rare.

Every year, the World Health Organisation (WHO), together with the International Union Against Cancer, puts forward ways to reduce the burden of this disease. But the battle is unequal, with different regions of the world not being equal in the face of cancer.

Any prevention policy cannot be implemented without accurate epidemiological studies and statistical analyses. Without epidemiological surveillance, it is impossible to implement a national or even regional plan to combat the most common digestive cancers.

In Algeria, a national network of registries was created in 2014 as part of the 2015-2019 cancer plan (strategic axis number 6). Its creation was reinforced by an order *(№22 of 18 February 2014)*, which institutionalized population registries in each wilaya. This has allowed the consolidation of existing registers and the establishment of wilayas that lacked them[10] .

This institutionalisation of registers has resulted in a large coverage of valid registers in 2015 at 68%. These registration tools have made it possible to have reliable incidence data, representative of the whole country, with the possibility of making projections for the coming years.

The 48 wilayas of the country are divided into three regional networks: East and South-East, Centre and South-Centre and West and South-West, coordinated by the National Network of Cancer Registries of Algeria (RNRCA). [11]

In 2015, according to the data of these 3 networks of the RNRCA, the total number of cases and the incidence are respectively 42720 and 106.8 / 100 000 inhabitants. Digestive cancers in Algeria represent a quarter of cancers in general. Colon and rectal cancer are in the lead; they represent 15% of all cancers.

In men, CRC (colorectal cancer) is in first place with a crude rate of 16.9/100,000 inhabitants; in women, however, it is in second place after breast cancer with a crude rate of 14.3/100,000 inhabitants. Stomach cancer ranks fifth in both sexes with 2111 cases. Hence the interest of a detailed epidemiological study of these important sites. The aim of this work is to make an epidemiological study on the incidence, the geographical distribution and the evolution of digestive cancers in the East and South East region of Algeria.

CHAPTER 1

DESCRIPTIVE EPIDEMIOLOGY OF DIGESTIVE CANCERS

1.1. Epidemiology of all digestive cancers :

To study the incidence of cancers, it is necessary to distinguish between incidence, which is the number of new cases of cancer diagnosed during a given period, and prevalence, which is the total number of cancer cases reported at a given time. Incidence can be further defined by morbidity, which indicates the number of cases of disease observed in a given population, or by deaths, which indicate mortality due to that disease.

1.1.1. In the world :

Data on the incidence of cancer worldwide are readily available and provide information on estimated morbidity and mortality for 2018. These projections are based on statistics from the **Globocan 2018** database, compiled by the *International Agency for* Research *on Cancer* (*IARC)* and global incidence data from Cancer Incidence in Five Continents (*CI5)* **(Figure 1).**

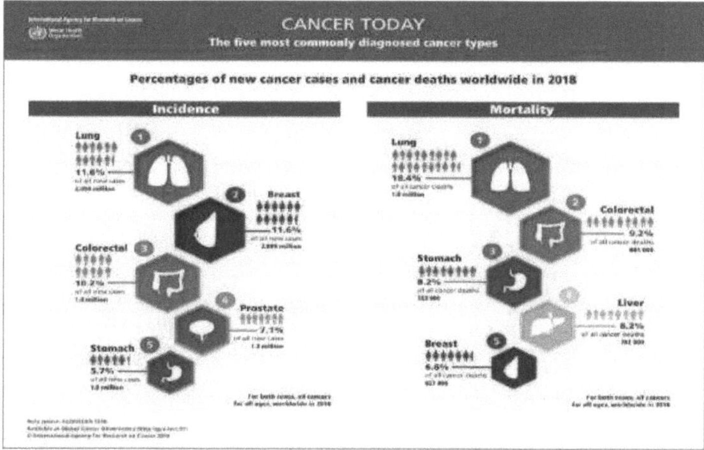

Source: Globocan 2018

Figure 1: Incidence and mortality data for the top 5 cancer sites in both sexes worldwide.

In 2002, the annual number of new cases of digestive cancers was 1,010,279 in men and 578,713 in women. Stomach cancer was among the most common malignancies worldwide, with 870,000 cases per year and 650,000 deaths. Developing countries account for 60% of cases. The highest incidences are found in East Asia and the Andean regions of South America.

For both sexes, stomach cancer ranks first among digestive cancers with an incidence rate of 12.3, followed by resophageal cancer with a rate of 7.7 and colon cancer with a rate of 7.1. This is followed by gallbladder and pancreatic cancer with an incidence rate of 2.6 and 1.9 respectively **(*Globocan*, 2002).**

In 2018, according to *Globocan* estimates, the top 5 digestive cancer sites (colon, rectum, stomach, liver, pancreas and resophagus) accounted for 26.3% of all cancers, or 4.8 million cases, and were responsible for 35.4% of these cases, or 3.4 million deaths[12] **(figure 3)**.

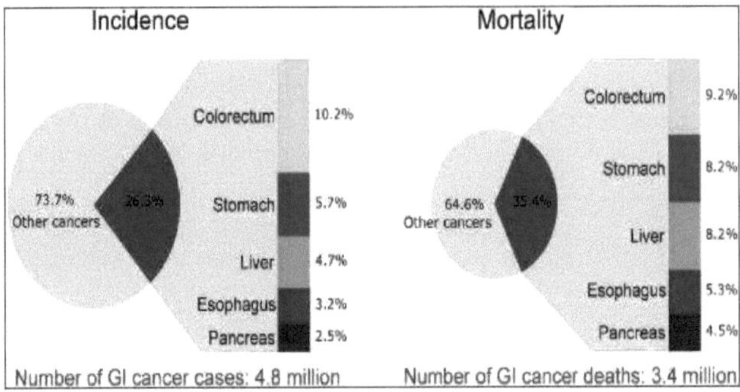

Source: Globocan 2018

Figure 2: Global burden of the 5 main types of digestive cancers, incidence and mortality.

Geographical and temporal variations in incidence and mortality are observed for the five types of gastrointestinal cancers. Cancers of the resophagus, stomach and liver are more common in Asia than in other parts of the world, while colorectal and pancreatic cancers are higher in Europe and North America. There is a uniform decrease in the incidence of gastric cancer, but an increasing incidence of colorectal cancer in areas previously with low incidence. Slight increases in liver and pancreatic cancer incidence are seen in some high-income regions.[12] **(Figure 3)**

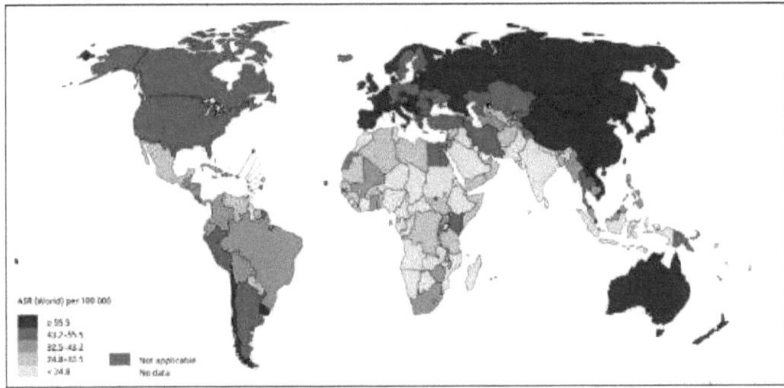

Source: Globocan 2018

Figure 3: Age-standardised incidence rates of digestive cancers worldwide in both sexes.

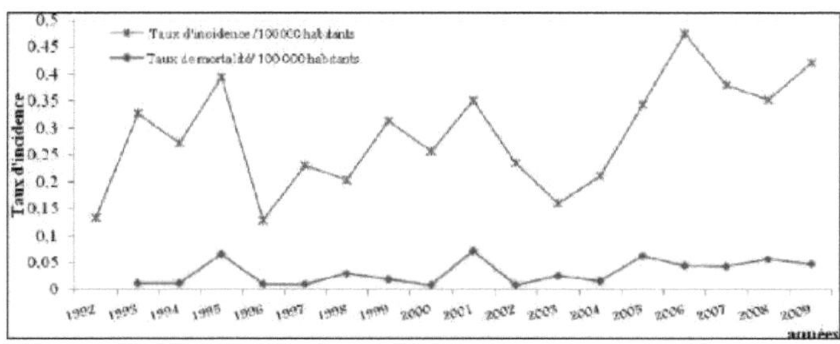

Source: DIGESTIVE CANCER IN NIGER, EUROPEAN SCIENTIFIC JOURNAL

Figure 4: Trend in incidence and mortality rates of digestive cancers in both sexes.

1.1.2. In Algeria :

According to *Globocan* estimates (2002), liver cancer ranked first among men, followed by colon and rectal cancer for both sexes. Stomach cancer was in third place and finally pancreatic and resophageal cancers appeared with low rates.

In 2012, digestive cancers represent about 25% of cancers in men and 17.5% of cancers in women. Colorectal cancer is ranked 2eme (about 50% of digestive cancers), stomach cancer is ranked 5eme (% of digestive cancers).

In women, cancers of the extrahepatic bile ducts (EABD), and in particular gallbladder cancer, occupy an important place.

In 2011, in Algiers, the number of new cases of digestive cancers was 1061 cases, i.e. a crude incidence rate of 32.8/100,000 inhabitants.

According to data from the Batna register published in CI5 volume 11 (2008 - 2012), digestive cancers represent 27.4% of cancers in men and 24.8% of cancers in women. For Setif, the standardised incidence of all digestive cancers is 21.7 per 100,000 inhabitants in men and 21.8 per 100,000 inhabitants in women.

1.2. Epidemiology of colorectal cancer

CRC is a major public health problem in developed countries because of its frequency and severity. Annually, nearly one million two hundred thousand cases are diagnosed with half a million deaths. CRCs rank third among cancers in terms of incidence and mortality.

1.2.1. In the world :

1.2.1.1. Incidence

Colon cancer is the fourth most common cancer site worldwide, while rectal cancer is the eighth most common. Worldwide, CRC is the third most diagnosed cancer, accounting for 10.2% of all diagnosed cancers[13, 14] .

According to *Globocan* 2018 data, approximately 1,096,000 new cases of colon cancer were diagnosed and approximately 704,000 new cases of rectal cancer.

Gender variations: CRC is more common in men and 3-4 times more common in developed countries; with an age-standardised incidence rate (ASR) for both sexes of 19.7/100,000 population (23.6 in men and 16.3 in women)[14]. While the ASR for men is 30.1/100,000 in high HDI (human development index) countries, it is 8.4 in low HDI countries (the same statistics for women are 20.9 and 5.9 respectively)[13].

Geographical variations: Globally, the highest incidence rates are found in Australia, New Zealand, Europe and North America, and the lowest rates are found in Africa and South-Central Asia[15] **(Figure 5).**

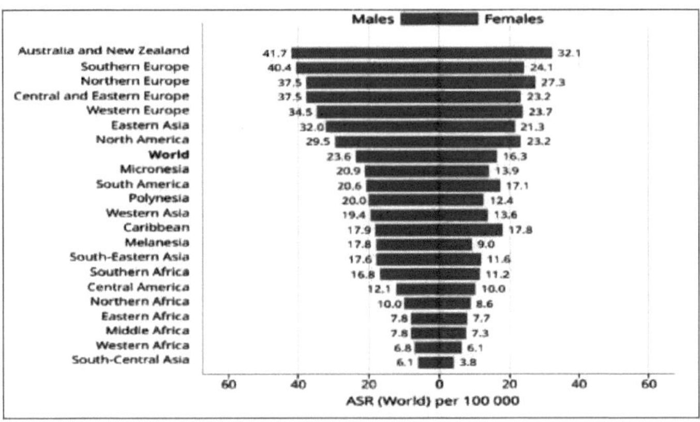

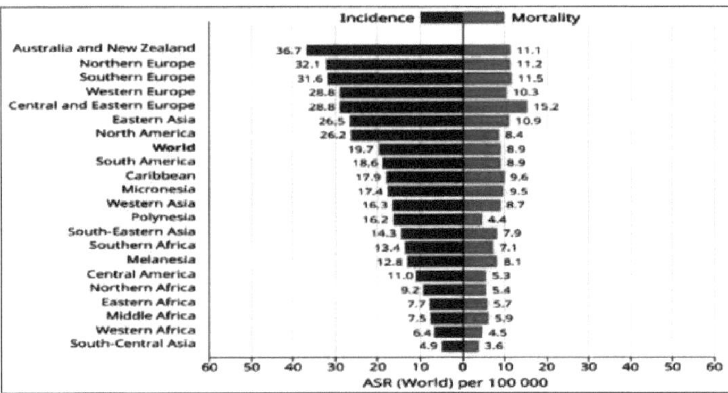

Source: Globocan 2018

Figure 5: Page-standardised incidence and mortality rates of colorectal cancer in both sexes.

These geographical differences appear to be attributable to differences in dietary habits, environmental exposures and genetic susceptibility.

Trend: In the United States, CRC incidence rates have been decreasing by about 2% per year[16,17]. Incidence rates in most other Western countries have remained stable or increased slightly during this period. In contrast, CRC incidence rates have increased rapidly in several historically low-risk areas, including Spain and a number of East Asian and European countries.

of the East [18, 19] **(Figure 6).**

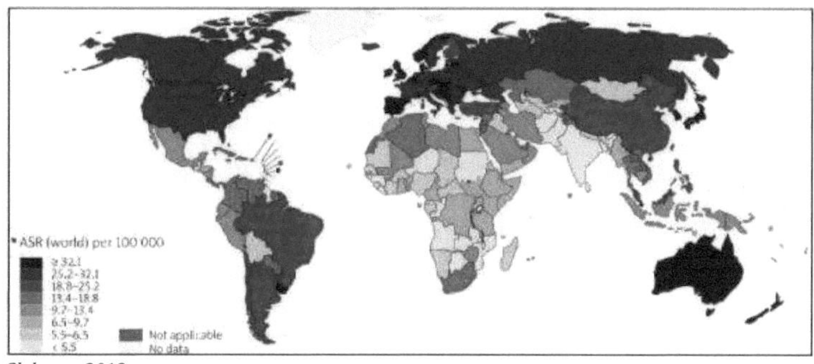

Source: Globocan 2018

Figure 6: Page-standardised incidence rate of colorectal cancer in 2018, both sexes combined.

Like Japan and Thailand, which are experiencing a rapid increase in CRC incidence. It has been rising steadily in Iran over the past 30 years(14) . Rates have more than doubled in Saudi Arabia since 1994, at the same time as rates have begun to rise in the Philippines.

On the other hand, CRC incidence rates have also been slowly increasing in Jordan, China, South Korea and Singapore. These are the regions where stomach and liver cancer frequencies are generally high **(Figure 7).**

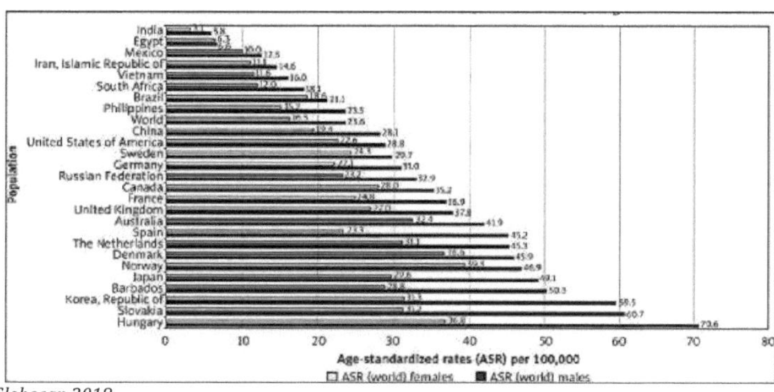

Source: Globocan 2018

Figure 7: Age-standardised incidence rates of CRC by country and sex.

In France

In 2018, the number of new cases of CRC is estimated at 43,336; 54% of which are in men. It is the third most common cancer in men and the second most common cancer in women among solid tumours. The standardised incidence rates are 34.0 cases per 100,000 person-years in men and 23.9 cases per 100,000 person-years in women (male/female ratio 1.4) **(Table 3, Figure 9)**(20) .

In Africa

In rural Africa, colon and rectal cancer is a rare disease; however, over the past 30 years, publications have reported an increase in the incidence of colorectal cancer in West Africa.

The crude incidence of CRC in sub-Saharan Africa is estimated at 4.04/100,000 population (4.38 males and 3.69 females).

Most of the available studies have shown an average age of between 43 and 46 years (maximum age 50-60 years), except in Ghana where the average age is 58 years (maximum age 70-80 years)[21] .

Table 1: Past incidence of colorectal cancer in sub-Saharan Africa

Country	Male/100K	Female/100,000	Period of study
Nigeria	2.5	3.2	1960-1969
Senegal	2.1	1.7	1969-1974
Gambia	1.5	0.5	1986-1988
Mali	23		1987-1988

Country	Cases/100,000	Period of study
Gambia	1.6	1988-1997
Mali	6.0	1988-1992
Guinea	61	1992-1995
Ivory Coast	2.4	1995-1997
Ghana	11.8	1997-2007
Nigeria	34	2000 till date

In 2018, according to *Globocan* estimates, CRC is the leading cancer. The highest incidence is observed in South Africa with 6937 new cases, followed by Niger with 6692 cases, Egypt with 5393 cases and Morocco with 4118 new cases.

1.2.1.2. Mortality :

CRC mortality rates have been gradually decreasing since the 1980s in the United States and many Western countries[22] . This improvement can be attributed to the detection and removal of colonic polyps, early detection of CRC and more effective primary and adjuvant therapy.

However, in the United States, the overall decline in mortality masks trends among young adults in particular. According to records derived from the *National Cancer Institute*'s *Surveillance Epidemiology and End Results* (*SEER*) database, CRC death rates per 100,000 population among people aged 20-54 years fell from 6.3 in 1970 to 3.9 in 2004, and then increased by 1% per year to 4.3 in 2014[23] **(Figure 8).**

In contrast to these data, mortality rates continue to rise in many countries with more limited health resources and infrastructure, particularly in Central and South America and Eastern Europe[22] .

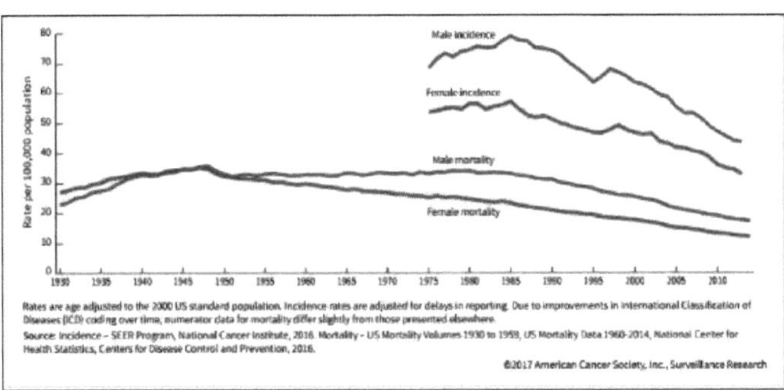

Figure 8: Trend in incidence (1975 - 2013) and mortality (1930 - 2014) by gender, USA.

In France: With 17,117 estimated deaths in 2018, 54% of which were men, CRC is the second most common cancer death in men and the third most common in women. The standardised mortality rates are 11.5 and 6.9 respectively (male/female ratio equal to 1.7)[20] **(Table 2).**

Table 2: Incidence and mortality in metropolitan France in 2018 *(table reproduced from national estimates of cancer incidence and mortality in metropolitan France between 1990 and 2018 volume 1: solid tumours/colon and rectum networks)*

	Number of cases	Gross rate	Standardised rate Europe	Standardised rate World
Incidence				
Male	23 216	73,7	50,9	34,0
Woman	20 120	60,0	35,0	23,9
Mortality				
Male	9209	29,2	18,4	11,5
Woman	1908	23,6	10,8	6,9

Figure 9: Colorectal cancer incidence and mortality rates in France by year (1990-2018).

1.2.2. In Algeria

In Algeria, the incidence of CRC has been rising steadily in recent years, due to the epidemiological transition and changes in lifestyle, to gradually reach that of Western countries. In 2012, the incidence was 3380 cases and the mortality was 2016 deaths. CRC is ranked second after breast cancer (8177 cases/year) in women and after lung cancer in men, with 1690 cases/year. The mortality rate in Algeria was $7.58/10^5$ and $6.7/10^5$ for men and women respectively (*Globocan*, 2012)

According to the cancer registry of the wilaya of Setif from 1986 to 2014, the incidence of CRC has increased by 5.7% in men and 5.5% in women[24] .
Over 81.7% of colorectal cancers occur in adults over 45 years of age.
The median age at diagnosis is 58 years **(Figure 10).**

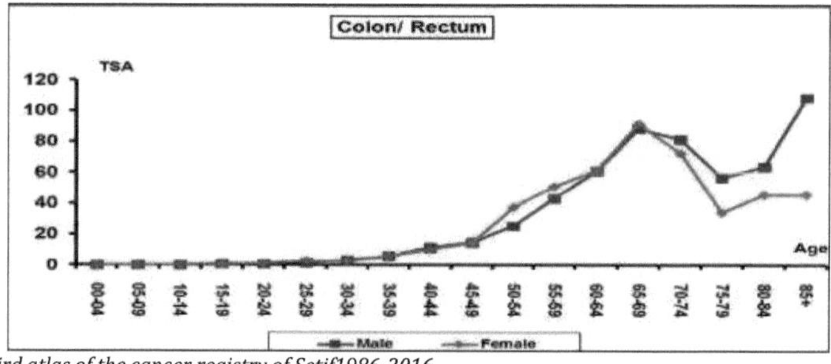

Source: Third atlas of the cancer registry of Setif1986-2016

Figure 10: Age-standardized CRC rates for both sexes, Setif 2016.
In 2015, the incidence rate is estimated at 13.7 in men and 14.0 in women per 100,000

inhabitants.

In 2018, the incidence of CRC is estimated at 2910 cases in men and 2627 cases in women ***(Globocan 2018***

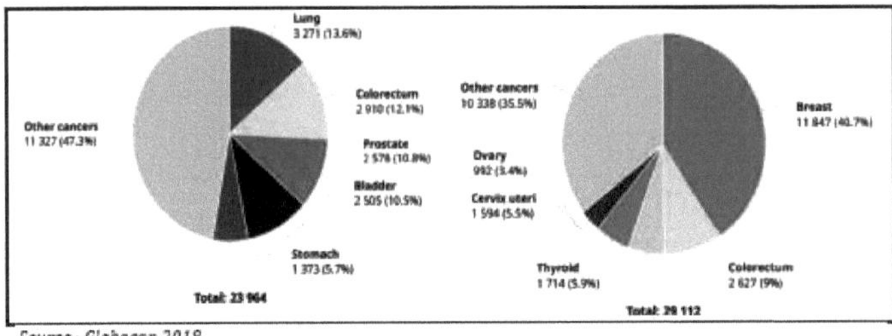

Figure 11: Incidence of colorectal cancer in Algeria in both sexes.
Source: Globocan 2018

Trend: According to the Setif Atlas, the incidence of colorectal cancer in men has increased significantly, *Annual Percent Change (APC)* +7.8 over the past decades, with the incidence rate rising from 2.6 in 1986 to 21.0 per 100,000 population in 2016.

In women, the incidence of colorectal cancer is constantly increasing (APC +6.5*). The standardised incidence has risen from 2.8 per 100,000 in 1986 to 21.4 per 100,000 in 2016 [25].

Homme **Femme**

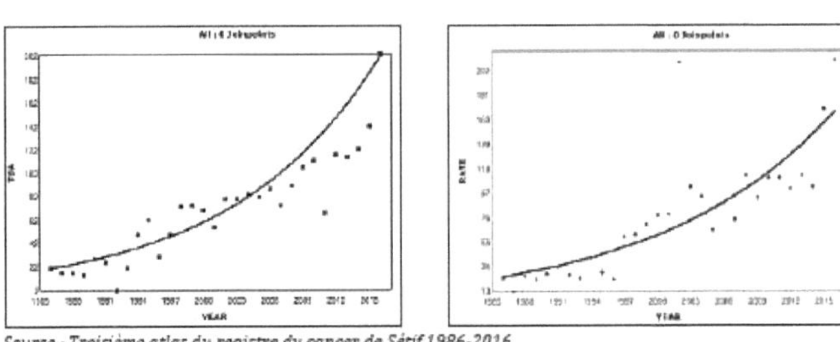

Figure 12: Trends in CRCs for both sexes 1986-2016, Setif willaya.
Source: Third atlas of the cancer registry of Setif1986-2016

1.2.3. Survival :

Improvements in CRC treatment and the introduction of better screening tests have led to a decrease in CRC-related mortality. Globally, the United States has one of the highest survival rates. Data collected by the US SEER programme reports that 61% of all patients treated for CRC (all stages and sites) survive five years[23] .

In Algeria, according to the Setif atlas 1986 - 2016: overall survival at 5 years (2000 - 2010)

Table 3: 5-year overall survival of colon and rectal cancers (2000 - 2010).

The overall survival o	**bserve of**	**colonic anchors**			
Year of survival	Number of cases	Number of deaths	Survival rate (SO)	Risk of error	[Int, Conf, 95%)
1	421	42	90,93%	0,0134	0,8792 - 0,9321

3	354	56	78,61%	0,0192	0,7456 - 0,8209
_5 154 29 71,12%				0,022	0,6654 - 0,7518

Overall Observed Survival of Rectal Cancers

Survival year	Number of cases	Number of deaths	Survival rate (SO)	Risk of error	[Int, Conf, 95%]
_1	311	42	88,12%	0,0172	0,8427-0,9108
3	246	59	71,13%	0,0243	0,6607-0,7558
J	127	16	66,14%	0,0256	0,6085-0,7088

According to the CONCORD 3 study, the 5-year survival rate of 788 cases from the 3 registers of : Setif, Annaba and Tlemcen, is 74.2% for the colon with a confidence interval of 65.7 - 82.7 and 67.3% for the rectum with a confidence interval of 58.0 - 76.5.

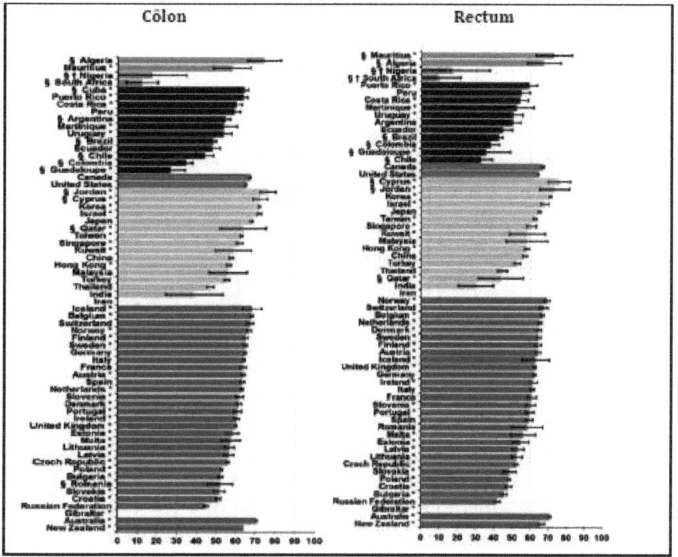

Figure 13: 5-year survival rates for CRC according to the CONCORD 3 study. 2010 - 2014

1.3. Epidemiology of gastric cancer

Although its incidence is steadily decreasing, stomach cancer remains one of the most common and deadliest cancers worldwide[13] .

According to *Globocan* 2018 data, gastric cancer is the third leading cause of cancer deaths worldwide. Approximately 1 in 12 cancer deaths is attributable to the gastric site.

1.3.1. In the world :

1.3.1.1. Incidence

More than one million cases of gastric cancer are diagnosed each year worldwide. Gastric cancer is the 5eme most diagnosed cancer in the world.[13] **(Figure 14)**. The incidence of distal gastric cancer is declining worldwide while that of cardiac cancer is stable.

Gender: Gastric cancer is more common in men. In developed countries, it is 2.2 times more likely to be diagnosed in men than in women. In developing countries, this ratio is 1.83[13].

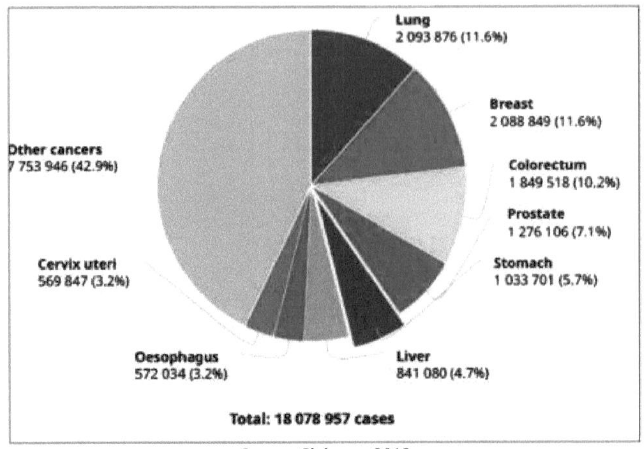

Source: Globocan 2018

Figure 14: Incidence of stomach cancer worldwide.

Age: Stomach cancer occurs most often in people over 55 years of age. Most people diagnosed with stomach cancer are between 60 and 70 years old.

Geographical variations

Stomach cancers are more frequently diagnosed in developed countries. The average incidence rate among countries with a medium-high HDI is 20 per 100,000, while the average rate among countries with a medium-low HDI is 6.6 per 100,000[13].

The incidence of gastric cancer varies greatly by region and culture. Incidence rates are highest in East and Central Asia and Latin America[26]. In East Asia, the average incidence of gastric cancer is 32.1 per 100,000 in men and 13.2 in women. In North America, the incidence is 5.6 per 100,000. The rate is lowest in North and East Africa, with only 4.7 per 100,000 men. North Korea has the highest incidence with almost 60 per 100,000 new cases per year in men. While incidence rates for women are lower (only 25 per 100,000 in Korea)[14] **(Figure 15).**

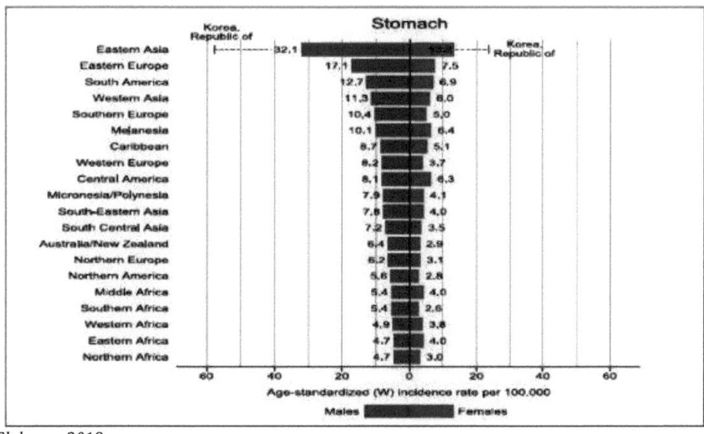

Source: Globocan 2018

Figure 15: Standardized incidence of gastric cancer worldwide in both sexes sexes.

[eme]In Europe, in 2014, there were approximately 140,000 newly diagnosed cases of gastric cancer, with gastric cancer representing the 6th most frequent cancer[27].

In France

[eme]In France, the number of new cases of gastric cancer diagnosed in 2014 is estimated at 6,500 cases, which places this cancer in 10th position, far behind lung, breast or colorectal cancers. Stomach cancers represent about 3% of all cancers and about 12% of digestive cancers[27].

In 2018, the number of new cases of stomach cancer in metropolitan France is estimated at 4,657, 65% of which are in men. The standardised incidence rates are respectively 6.3 cases per 100,000 person-years for men and 2.7 cases per 100,000 person-years for women (male/female ratio equal to 2.3).

The median age at diagnosis in 2018 is 71 and 75 for men and women respectively[20].

1.3.1.2. Mortality

Gastric cancer was the most common cause of cancer-related deaths worldwide until the mid-1990s. Gastric cancer is responsible for 783,000 deaths each year, making it the third most deadly cancer in men **(Figure 16)**, with 8.3% of cancer deaths attributable to this cancer[13].

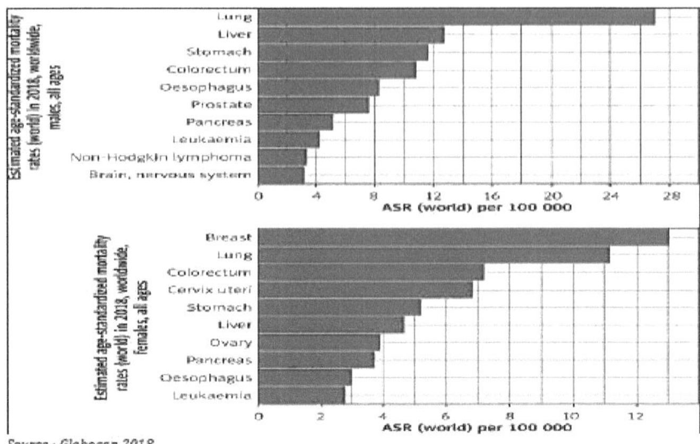

Source: Globocan 2018

Figure 16: Standardised mortality rates for gastric cancer by Page in both sexes in the world in 2018.

Mortality from gastric cancer is highest in men. Mortality rates are high in East and Central Asia and Latin America (the same high incidence regions)[26] **(Figure 17).**

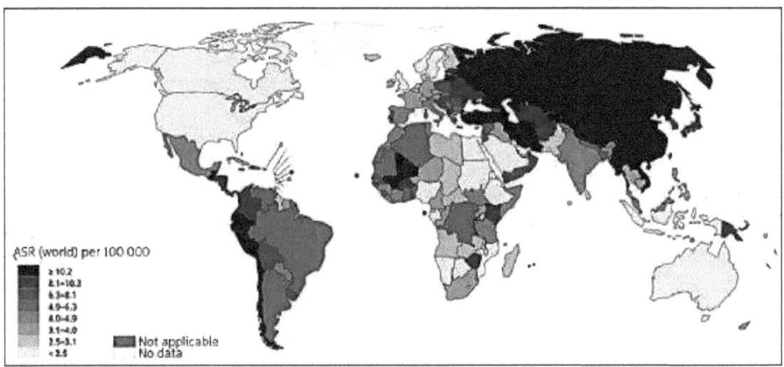

Source: Globocan 2018

Figure 17: Age-standardised mortality rates for stomach cancer (worldwide) in both sexes.

emeemeIn Europe, in 2014, there were approximately 140,000 new cases of gastric cancer diagnosed, making it the 6th most frequent cancer and the 4th leading cause of cancer deaths with 107,000 deaths per year[27] .

In France, the estimated number of deaths from stomach cancer in 2018 was 4,272, 65% of which were in men. The standardised mortality rates are respectively 3.9 and 1.5 per 100,000 (male/female ratio equal to 2.6).
The average age at death in 2018 is 73 for men and 79 for women[20].

1.3.2. In Algeria

Algeria is one of the low-risk countries for gastric cancer, with a declining incidence (from 9.4 per 100,000 population in men and 6.9 per 100,000 population in women in 2011 to an estimated 7.1 per 100,000 population in men and 4.3 per 100,000 population in women in 2018) **(Figure 18).**

It ranks 2eme among digestive cancers and 5eme among all cancers.

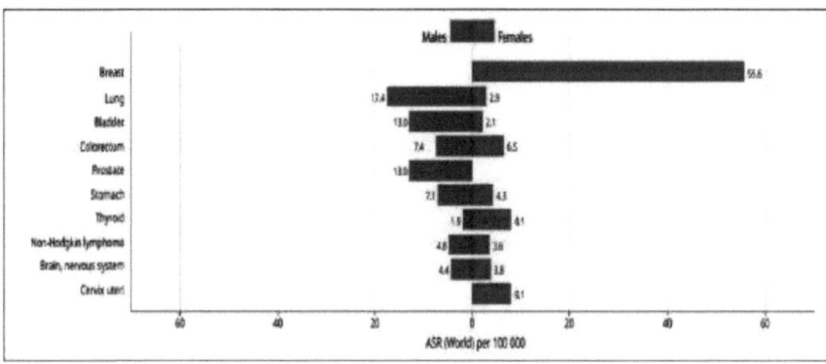

Source: Globocan 2018

Figure 18: Estimated ASR of incidence of the main cancers in Algeria.

In Setif during the period 2011-2016, 375 cases were recorded with a crude incidence of 4.2 in men and 3.4 in women, which corresponds to standardised rates of 6.0 and 4.4 respectively. Stomach cancer affects men 1.2 times more than women.

87% of stomach cancers occur in subjects over 45 years of age, and increase progressively to reach a maximum between 60-69 years of age and a second peak is recorded from 80 years of age, 73.1% are adenocarcinomas.

The incidence of stomach cancer has decreased very significantly (APC -3.1*)[24] .

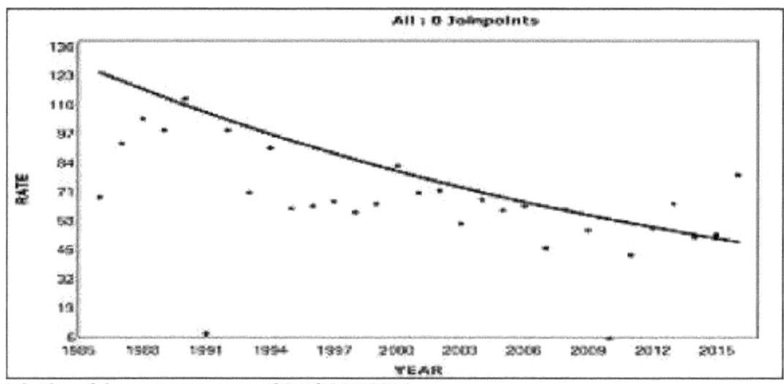

Source: Third atlas of the cancer registry of Setif1986-2016

Figure 19: Trends in male gastric cancer 1986-2016, wilaya of Setif.

1.3.3. Survival

In the USA, the 5-year survival rate for gastric cancer is 31%. The average survival rates reflect the fact that most cases diagnosed are already metastatic. The 5-year survival rate for pre-metastatic diagnosis is 67% [28].

In the UK, the 5-year survival rate is 19% and the 10-year survival rate is 15%. These rates show a clear improvement in the treatment of gastric cancer. For the period 1971-1972 in the UK, the 5-year survival rate was 5.3% and the 10-year survival rate was 4.1%[29] .

The average 5-year survival rate in Europe is 26%, higher than in the UK but lower than in the USA. The highest survival rate in Europe is in Iceland, which reports a 5-year survival rate of 42% for women [29].

In Algeria, according to the Atlas de Setif 1986 - 2016: overall survival at 5 years (2000 - 2010)

Table 4: 5-year overall survival for gastric cancer (2000 - 2010).

Overall Observed Survival of Stomach Cancers

Year of survival	Number of cases	Number of deaths	Survival rate (SO)	Risk of error	[Int, Conf, 95%]
1	246	153	61,63%	0,0244	0,5666-0,6620
3	79	116	28,05%	0,0243	0,2339-0,3288
5	37	21	19,47%	0,0231	0,1517-0,2419

According to the CONCORD 3 study, the 5-year survival rate of 385 cases from the 3 registries: Setif, Annaba and Tlemcen is 41.6% with a confidence interval between (35.5 - 47.7).

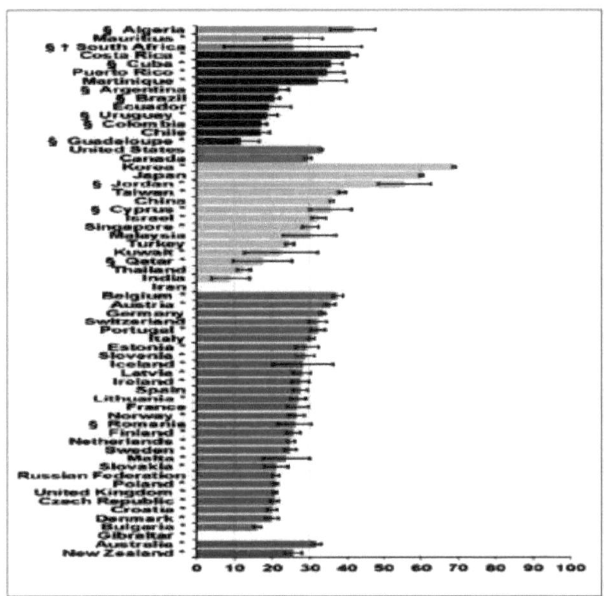

Figure 20 : 5-year relative survival rate for stomach cancer according to the CONCORD 3 study. 2010 - 2014.

1.4. Epidemiology of biliary tract cancers

Cholangiocarcinoma (CC) is a malignant neoplasm of the bile ducts representing 3% of gastrointestinal tumours[30] . It is the second most common primary liver tumour, accounting for 10-25% of primary liver tumours worldwide[30,31] . Anatomically, CC can be classified as intrahepatic or extrahepatic[32] .

CC rarely occurs before the age of 40[31,33] . Men have a higher incidence than women[34] with ratios between 1.2-1.5. The incidence of CC varies considerably by geographical region, due to variations in risk factors.

Gallbladder cancer

According to *Globocan* 2018 data, gallbladder cancer is the 22eme most common cancer but the 17eme deadliest cancer worldwide[13] .

1.4.1. In the world :

1.4.1.1. Incidence

Gender: Gallbladder cancer is the only digestive cancer that is more common in women. In 2018, the estimated incidence was 97,000 for men and 122,000 for women. However, the standardised incidence rate according to Page for women is 2.4 (per 100,000), and 2.2 for men *(Globocan)*.

Geographical variations: Incidence rates are highest in Eastern Europe, East Asia and Latin America. The incidence in the USA is lower than worldwide, with a rate of 1.4 per 100,000 in women and 0.8 in men[1 4, 35] **(Figure 21).**

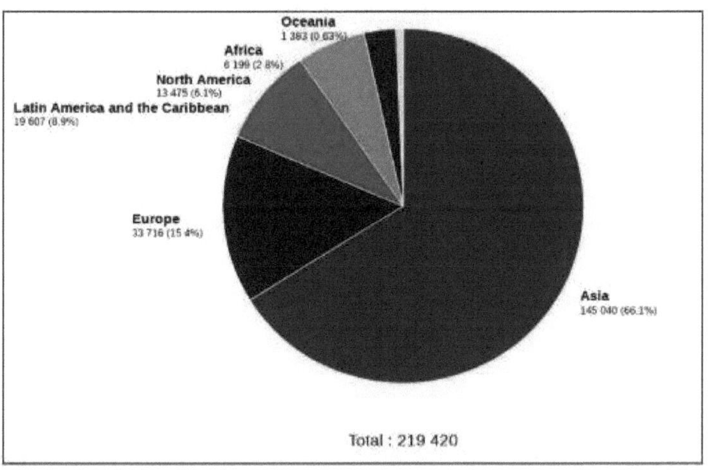

<u>Source: Globocan 2018</u>

Figure 21: Incidence of gallbladder cancer worldwide.

The countries with the highest ASR rates per 100,000 males in 2018 are Bolivia (12.8), Thailand (9.0), Republic of Korea (8.4), Chile (6.6) and Nepal (6.0). The countries with the five highest ASRs per 100,000 women in 2018 are Bolivia (15.1), Chile (11.7), Bangladesh (7.3), Nepal (7.3) and Peru (6.0) [14].

In France, the estimated number of new cases of gallbladder and extrahepatic biliary tract cancer in 2018 is 2,965, 52% of which are in men. The ASR rates are 2.1 cases per 100,000 person-years for men and 1.4 cases per 100,000 person-years for women (male to female ratio 1.5). The median age at diagnosis is 72 years for men and 78 years for women[20] .

1.4.1.2. Mortality

Gallbladder cancer mortality accounts for 1.7% of all cancer deaths. Approximately 165,000 people died of gallbladder cancer in 2018. Of these, approximately 70,000 were men and 95,000 were women.

The standardised mortality rate is 1.6/100,000 for men and 1.8 for women[13] .

Worldwide, age-standardised mortality rates for this location for both sexes (per 100,000) are highest in Central and Eastern Europe (Slovakia 3.2, Hungary 2.5, Poland 2.2), East Asia (Republic of Korea 4.1, Japan 3.3, Cambodia 2.6) and Latin America (Bolivia 10.6, Chile 5.4, Peru

3.1). Bolivia had the highest mortality rate[13,14]. A few countries, including Japan and South Korea, had higher mortality for men than for women.

1.4.2. In Algeria

Cancer of the extrahepatic bile ducts is a relatively common location, particularly in women.

emeGallbladder cancer is the most common cancer of the bile ducts, and the third most common digestive cancer in Algeria after colorectal and stomach cancer.

In 2012, in Algiers the standardised incidence rates were 2.1 and 4.2 for men and women respectively.

In Setif, between 2011 and 2016, 168 cases of biliary cancer were recorded, corresponding to a standardised incidence per 100,000 inhabitants of 3.4 in women and 1.4 in men. This pathology affects women 2.4 times more than men. 92.6% of biliary tract cancers occur in women from the age of 45 years, increasing progressively with age and reaching a maximum between 60-64 years, with a second peak at 85 years. The median age is 64.4 years[24].

1.5. Epidemiology of pancreatic cancer

Pancreatic cancer has the poorest prognosis in any region of the world, with 330,300 deaths per year and an estimated global prevalence and incidence of 211,500 and 337,900 cases respectively in 2012[36].
In the United States and other developed countries, pancreatic cancer is the fourth leading cause of cancer-related deaths[37].
In Europe, in 2012, the incidence rate of pancreatic cancer for both sexes was 10.1/100,000, with an attributable mortality of 9.9/100,000 deaths[38].

1.5.1. In the world

1.5.1.1. Incidence

The incidence of pancreatic cancer varies between regions and populations. In 2018, 458,918 new cases of pancreatic cancer were recorded worldwide, representing 2.5% of all cancers[39].

Geographical variations: The ASR of incidence is highest in Europe (7.7 per 100,000 people) and North America (7.6 per 100,000 people), followed by Oceania (6.4 per 100,000 people). The lowest rate was observed in Africa with an estimated incidence of 2.2 per 100,000 people[13].

Sex: A slight difference in the incidence of pancreatic cancer between the sexes as well as different geographical distributions have been observed. It is more common in men (5.5 per 100,000, 243,033 cases) than in women (4.0 per 100,000, 215,885 cases). In men, the risk of developing pancreatic cancer is high in Central and Eastern Europe. The regions with the highest incidence of pancreatic cancer in women are Western Europe (7.2), North America (6.5), Northern Europe and Australia/New Zealand (also: 6.4). The regions with the lowest risk (less than 1.0 per 100,000) of developing pancreatic cancer in women are East Africa and South East Asia. [39]**(Figure 22)**

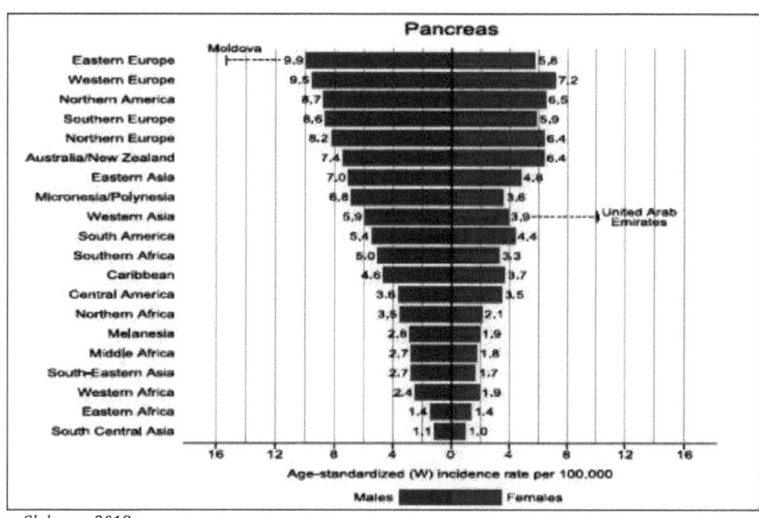

Source: Globocan 2018

Figure 22: Standardised incidence of pancreatic cancer worldwide in both sexes.

Age: The incidence rate for both sexes increases with age[39,40] . Pancreatic cancer is rarely diagnosed before the age of 55, and can be defined as a disease of the elderly as the highest incidence is reported in people over 70[40] .

France: In 2018, the number of new cases of pancreatic cancer is estimated at 14,184, 51% of which are in men. Pancreatic cancer accounts for 18% of digestive cancers, of which it is the third most common cancer in men and the second most common in women. The standardised incidence rates are of 11.0 cases per 100,000 person-years in men and 7.7 cases per 100,000 person-years in women (sex ratio equal to 1.4)[20] .

1.5.1.2. Mortality

International mortality rates for pancreatic cancer vary widely around the world. In 2018, the highest mortality rates were recorded in Western Europe (7.6 per 100,000 population), Central and Eastern Europe (7.3), followed by Northern Europe and North America (also 6.5). The lowest rate was reported in East Africa (1.4), South-East Asia and West Africa (also: 2.1)[13] **(Figure 23)**. More than half of pancreatic cancer deaths occurred in the most developed countries (52.3% or 226,272 deaths). The mortality rate from pancreatic cancer in both men and women increases with age, and almost 90% of all deaths occur after age 55[13] .

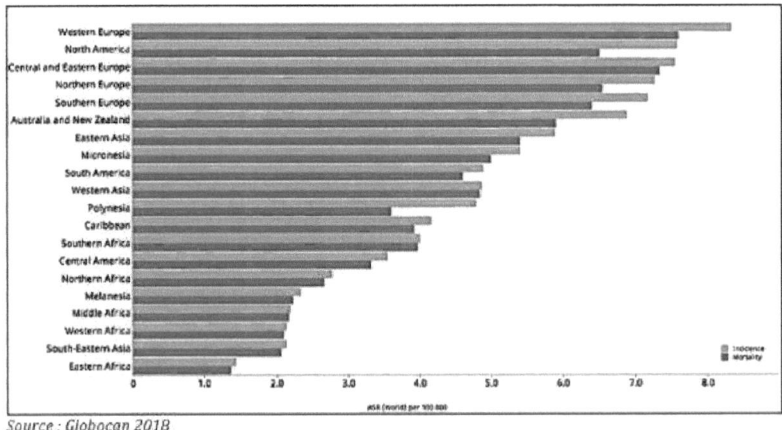

Source : Globocan 2018

Figure 23: Standardised incidence and mortality of pancreatic cancer worldwide.

In France, with an estimated 11,456 deaths in 2018, 50% of which were in men, pancreatic cancer is the fifth most common cause of cancer deaths in men and the fourth most common in women. The mortality rates are 8.2 and 5.5 per 100 000 person-years respectively (male/female ratio equal to 1.5)[20] .

1.5.2. In Algeria

In Algeria, pancreatic cancer has a low incidence (3 to 4 per 100,000 inhabitants) and is more frequent in men (sex ratio, between 1.25 and 1.75), and occurs from the age of 50 to 55 years. According to the Algiers tumour register, the incidence of pancreatic cancer is estimated at 3.2/105 inhabitants for men and 1.7/105 inhabitants for women. Two thirds of cases are diagnosed after the age of 65.

1.5.3. Survival

The prognosis of pancreatic cancer is poor, with an overall survival rate of only 3.5% at 5 years. Several causes are commonly accepted to attest to its poor prognosis:

- late diagnosis due to often non-specific symptoms or a completely clinically silent phase at the beginning of the disease;
- an aggressiveness responsible for a rapid local and general extension by lymphatic and

nerve pathways as well as for metastases sometimes early;

- Rapid invasion of the vascular axes: given the anatomical location of the pancreas. '
- The difficulty and delicacy of pancreatic surgery which is a source of significant morbidity and mortality.
- Finally, the anatomical situation of the pancreas makes it a difficult organ to visualise by imaging.

From 2014 to 2018, the 5-year survival rate for pancreatic cancer increased from 6% to 9%, showing that progress is being made and that there is an urgent need to further improve survival. Indeed, to date, pancreatic cancer remains one of the most lethal malignancies, with a poor prognosis and a mortality/incidence ratio of 94% (13).

1.6. Epidemiology of liver cancer

Primary liver cancer is the sixth most frequently diagnosed cancer and the fourth most common cause of cancer death worldwide, with an estimated 841,000 cases (9.3 cases per 100,000 person-years) and 78,000 deaths (8.5 deaths per 100,000 person-years) in 2018. It is more common in men than in women[(13)] .

The two main histological types are hepatocellular carcinoma, which accounts for about 75% of all liver cancer cases, and intrahepatic CC (about 12-15%)[(41)] . The incidence rates of liver cancer vary from 5.1 per 100,000 person-years in Europe to 17.7 per 100,000 person-years in East Asia (14).

1.6.1. Incidence and mortality

Geographic variations: According to *Globocan* 2018 data, primary liver cancer resulted in an estimated 781,631 deaths at an age-standardised mortality rate of 8.5/100,000, and 841,080 cases were diagnosed in 2018. Men account for 596,574 cases and 548,375 deaths, more than twice as many as primary liver cancer in women (cases: 244,506; deaths: 233,456). The overall age-standardised incidence rate was 9.3/100,000 in 2018, ranging from Morocco (1.1/100,000) to Mongolia (93.7/100,000). There was also remarkable variation in terms of standardised mortality rates, ranging from 1/100,000 in Nepal to 75.4/100,000 in Mongolia. East Asia was the leading region contributing 55.6% of global cases and 54.7% of global deaths[(13)] **(Figure 24, 25).**

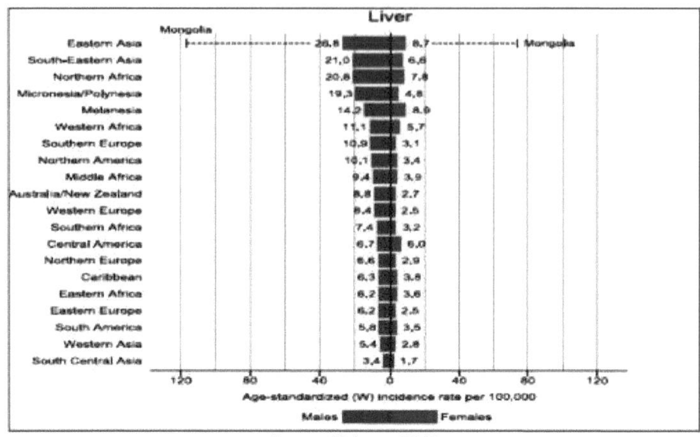

Source: Globocan 2018

Figure 24: Standardized incidence of liver cancer worldwide in both sexes sexes.

Gender and age: Liver cancer is the fifth most common cancer in men and the seventh in women(42) . The worldwide incidence is between 250,000 and 1,000,000 new cases per year with a male to female ratio of about 4. Its occurrence peaks at around 70 years of age, rarely before the age of 40 ,(4243) .

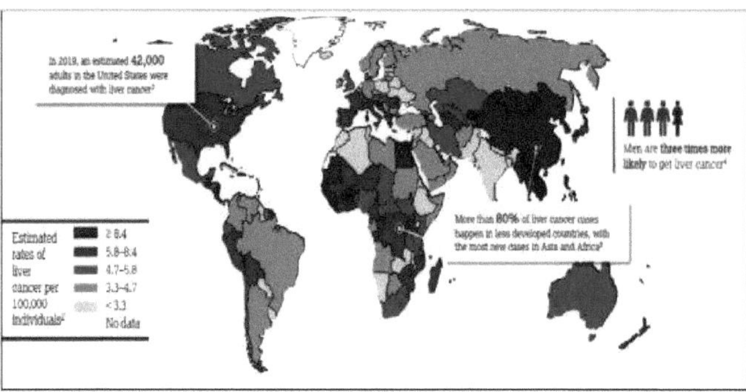

Source: Globocan 2018

Figure 25: Age-standardised incidence rate of primary liver cancer worldwide.

In France, the incidence of the disease has also been rising sharply over the past 20 years. The number of cases has risen from 1,800 in 1980 to around 10,700 in 2018. Liver cancer is now the 10eme most common site of the disease and represents 13% of digestive cancers. The annual incidence rates per 100,000 standardised people are 12.5 in men and 2.9 in women. It is therefore five times more common in men. The average age of discovery of the disease is 62 years(20) .

1.6.2. Survival

For the 44% of people diagnosed early, the 5-year survival rate is 34%. If there is a locoregional metastasis, the 5-year survival rate is 12%. If the cancer has spread to a distant part of the body, the 5-year survival rate is 3%. If surgery is possible, this usually results in higher survival rates at all stages of the disease(44) .

1.7. Epidemiology of resophageal cancer

Incidence and mortality

There is a wide disparity in the incidence of esophageal cancer worldwide(45) . Resophageal cancer is the 6eme cause of cancer deaths and the 8eme most common location in the world. Five-year survival is approximately 15% to 25% and the best outcomes are related to early diagnosis. (46)

Resophageal squamous cell carcinoma is the predominant histological type worldwide. However, at present, in countries such as the United States, Australia, the United Kingdom and Western Europe (Finland, France, Norway), there is a predominance of adenocarcinoma, with squamous cell carcinoma taking second place(46 ,47) . Turkey, Iran, Kazakhstan and northern and central China, with an estimated 100+ cases of resophageal squamous cell carcinoma per 100,000 person-years. Another area with a high incidence of squamous cell carcinoma is South East Africa.

In European countries such as the UK, France or Norway, the age-standardised incidence has increased by 39.6% for men and 37.5% for women over the last five years(46) . There is also a significant difference between the gender distributions; the incidence of the disease is approximately 2-4 times higher in men than in women ,(4849) . Overall, mortality rates follow a major parallelism with incidence rates in each country(46) .

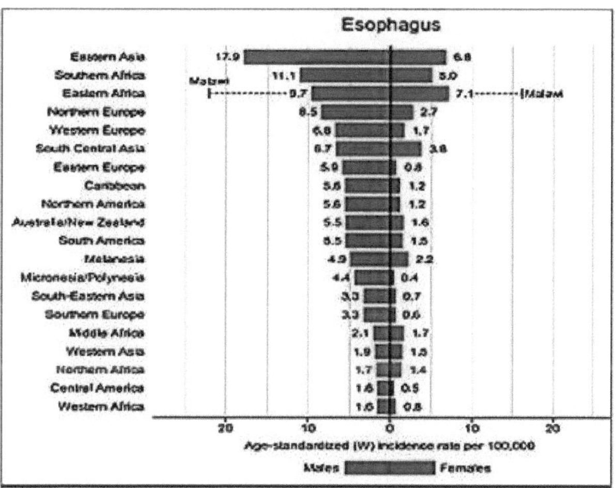

Source: Globocan 2018

Figure 26: Age-standardised incidence and mortality rates of resophageal cancers in both sexes worldwide.

In France, in 2018, the number of new cases of resophageal cancer is estimated at 5,445, 78% of which are in men. The standardised incidence rates in the world are 6.8 cases per 100,000 person-years for men and 1.5 cases per 100,000 person-years for women (male/female ratio equal to 4.5).
The number of deaths from resophageal cancer in 2018 is estimated at 3,725, of which 77% were in men. The mortality rates are 4.3 and 1.0 per 100,000 person-years for men and women respectively (male/female ratio 4.3). The median ages at diagnosis and death in 2018 are 67 and

69 years for men and 70 and 73 years for women respectively[20].

1.8. Epidemiology of small bowel cancer

Graft bowel cancer is a rare tumour, accounting for less than 5% of all cancers of the digestive tract[50,51], and has multiple histological forms. Adenocarcinoma is the most common histological form, followed by neuroendocrine tumours, sarcomas and lymphomas[50, 52, 53].

Incidence and mortality

International data show that the incidence is higher in North America, Western Europe and Oceania than in Asia[54, 55].

In 2018, there were approximately 10470 cases of small bowel cancer in the United States. This represents an incidence rate of 2.3 per 100,000 people. These cases also represent only 0.6% of all cancer cases in the US that year[54].

The UK has a comparable rate of bowel cancer cases, with an incidence of 3.1/100,000 in men and 2.2/100,000 in women[56].

Age and sex: Incidence increases after age 40 for all histological subtypes, with carcinomas and carcinoid tumours increasing much more rapidly than lymphomas. Rates stabilise after age 70 for carcinoid tumours, while sarcoma incidence increases more slowly than the other three types and stabilises after age 60[55]. Men have higher incidence rates than women, overall and for all histological subtypes of graft bowel cancer in most countries[57, 58, 59].

In France, in 2018, there were an estimated 1,746 new cases of graft bowel cancer, 56% of which occurred in men. The standardised incidence rates are 1.6 cases per 100,000 person-years in men and 1.0 case per 100,000 person-years in women (male/female ratio equal to 1.6). The median age at diagnosis is 68 years for men and 70 years for women[20].

Mortality from tumours of the grafted bowel is 0.5/100,000 for men and 0.3 for women in the USA. The median age of death is 72 years. An estimated 1450 Americans died of graft bowel cancer in 2018, which represented 0.2% of all cancer deaths. While the incidence has been increasing, the average mortality has remained at 0.4 since 1976[54].

Meanwhile, mortality is twice as high in the UK, with rates of 1.0 and 0.7 for men and women respectively. Since the 1970s, mortality from grafted bowel cancer has increased by 37% in the UK. It is highest in men and women in Scotland, and lowest in Wales for men and Northern Ireland for women. The most common age of death from transplanted bowel cancer is 85-89 years, almost a decade older than the UK life expectancy[56].

CHAPTER 2

ANALYTICAL EPIDEMIOLOGY OF DIGESTIVE CANCERS

2.1. Risk factors for colorectal cancer

2.1.1. Subjects at risk

The population can be classified into three groups according to their risk level[60, 61]:

- An average risk group (75%):

- All subjects over 50 years of age of both sexes, even without digestive disorders, will be offered a blood test in the stool by "*Hemoccult*", every two years. A colonoscopy will be performed in case of a positive test result.
- **Sporadic CRC** Sporadic CRC has no obvious hereditary background and represents the majority of CRCs (85-90%). Patients affected by this disease do not have germline genetic mutations but acquire mutations responsible for tumour development throughout their lives through exposure to various chemical, viral, bacterial or dietary cancerogens.

- A high risk group (20%):

- A personal history of adenoma larger than 1 cm or colorectal cancer.
- Family history of advanced adenoma (> 1 cm or large) or colorectal cancer of a first-degree relative (father, mother, brother, sister) under 60 years of age, two or more family histories of first-degree relatives with CRC regardless of age.
- Patients with a history of extensive and long-standing inflammatory bowel disease such as ulcerative colitis (left colon > 15 years), pancolitis > 10 years or *Crohn's* disease.
- Acromegalia[62].

- A very high risk group (5%):

- In hereditary forms, this group includes subjects with familial polyadenomatosis (FAP), accounting for less than 1% of CRCs, as well as carriers of hereditary non-polyposis colorectal cancers, HNPCC (*Hereditary NonPolyposis Colorectal Cancer)* syndrome, also known as *Lynch* syndrome, accounting for 1-5% of CRCs.

These are hereditary cancers without polyposis and a genetic diagnosis is now possible in these families[61, 63].

2.1.2. Non-modifiable risk factors for CRC :

2.1.2.1. Individuals :

- **Age:** Colorectal cancer is a cancer that increases in frequency with age. Before the age of 40, CRC is rare. The risk increases from the age of 50 onwards and increases up to the age of 80. 94% of colorectal cancers occur in people over 50 (Institut National du Cancer **INCa).** 90% of colorectal cancers are rarely diagnosed before the age of 45. The average age at diagnosis is 70[64]. In France the average age of detection is 70 for men and 73 for women in 2012[65].

In the population aged 50-74 years, with no other risk factor than age, the risk of developing colorectal cancer is estimated at 3.5%[60].

- **Gender:** CRC affects men more than women with a sex ratio of 1.47, this excess risk is probably related to differences in exposure to risk factors such as lifestyle, diet, smoking, obesity and exposure to restrogens[14] .

2.1.2.2. Personal history

- **Personal history of colorectal adenoma** :

In a man or woman who has had an adenoma resected, the risk of a new colorectal adenoma is increased by a factor of 4 if the adenoma has a villous structure or is >10 mm in diameter, and by a factor of 7 if the adenomas are multiple[60] , if it is an advanced colorectal adenoma, the risk of developing CRC is increased by a factor of 2 (*Odds-Ratio* OR= **1.77** [1.17-2.66]) ***Freedman A, et al.JCO 2009.***

- **Personal history of colorectal cancer:**

In a man or woman who has had a complete resection of colorectal cancer, the risk of a new CRC is significantly higher in the first 5 years after treatment of the initial colorectal cancer. 1.5% metachronous cancer at 5 years (Relative Risk RR = 6.8 [2.7-22]) with a median time to onset = 18 months. ***GreenR,et al.Ann Inter Med 2002.***

- **Inflammatory bowel diseases :**

- People with ulcerative colitis and Crohn's disease have an 8 to 30 times greater risk of developing early colon or rectal cancer[66] , especially when the entire bowel is affected and the condition is chronic[67, 68, 69]

- Other cancers :

- Women with breast, ovarian or uterine cancer also have a moderate excess risk of developing a new cancer in the colon or rectum[64] .

2.1.2.3. Genetic and family factors

- **Family history of colorectal cancer**

In a man or woman with a family history of colorectal cancer, the risk of cancer depends on the number of affected relatives, the age of the index case(s) and the degree of relationship to the index case(s)[60] .

- **Risk factor related to a genetic mutation**

The hereditary forms of colorectal cancer can be grouped into two main entities: polyposis and non-polyposis.

Non-polyposis forms: Non-polyposis forms are dominated by Lynch syndrome, which accounts for about 3% of colorectal cancer patients. These are often families where several people develop colorectal cancer.

In these families, colorectal cancer most often occurs at an earlier age (before 50 years) than in the general population. In patients with Lynch syndrome, the transition from a (benign) polyp to a (malignant) tumour occurs much more rapidly than in patients with non-hereditary colorectal cancer, and its transmission is autosomal dominant[70, 71] . This syndrome is defined by the presence of all the Amsterdam criteria (see Appendix IV).

The risk of CRC in people with Lynch syndrome is estimated at 80%[60] .

Polyposis forms :

- Familial Adenomatous Polyposis: FAP is characterized by the presence of hundreds or thousands of adenomas in the colon or rectum and is linked to two types of mutations:

- An autosomal dominant inheritance with high penetrance of a mutation in the *Anaphase Promoting Complex* gene.
- An autosomal recessive transmission of the MUTYH gene mutation.

Without treatment, the risk of colorectal cancer is 100%[(60)].

-Hamartomatous polyposis: Hamartomatous polyposis is a very rare condition with an estimated prevalence of 1/100,000 births. The three known entities are characterized by autosomal dominant inheritance and correspond to **Juvenile Polyposis, Peutz-Jeghers Syndrome and Cowden's Disease**[(70, 72)].

2.1.3. Modifiable risk factors

Colorectal cancer is linked to lifestyle, obesity, alcohol consumption, smoking, and high consumption of processed or red meat. All of these factors increase the risk of developing this type of cancer, while daily exercise and a varied diet (fruit, vegetables, cereals, milk) could reduce its incidence[(73)].

Aspirin and anti-inflammatory drugs have a protective effect on the development of colorectal cancer and adenomas. Studies have been conducted and others are underway that clarify the benefit of prevention that will not be offset by the side effects of aspirin (see chapter on prevention)[(74)].

Table 5: CRC risk and protective factors, CRC screening IARC 2019.

Risk factor	Categories	RR (<	15% CI)	Reference
Consumption of processed meat	Per 50 g/day	1.16(1.08-1.26)		WCRF/AICR (2017)
Alcohol consumption	Per 10 g/day of ethanol1	.07 (1.05-1.08)		WCRF/AICR (2017)
Body fatness	Per 5 kg/m² of BMI	Colorectum: 1.05(1.03-1.07)		WCRF/AICR (2017)
		Colon: 1.07(1.05-1.09)		
		Rectum: 1.02(1.01-1.04)		
Abdominal fatness	Per 10 cm of waist circumference 1.02 (1.01-1.03)			WCRF/AICR (2017)
Tobacco smoking	Never smokers	1.00		IARC (2012)
	Current smokers	1.15(1.00-1.32)		
	Former smokers	1.20 (1.04-1.38)		
Attained adult height	Per 5 cm	1.05 (1.02-1.07)		WCRF/AICR (2017)
Sex[1]	Female		1.00	Ferlay et al (2018a)
	Male		1.47	
Age	45-49 yr		1.00	Ferlay et al. (2018a)
	50-54 yr		1.75	
	55-59 yr		2.85	
	60-64 yr		4.33	
	65-69 yr		6.30	
	>70 yr		10.29	
BMI, body mass index; CI, confidence interval; RR, relative risk; yr, years. [1] Calculated by the Working Group from GLOBOCAN 2018 incidence figures.				
Protective factor		Categories	RR (95% CI)	Reference
Consumption of dietary fibre		Per 10 g/day	0.91 (0.88-0.94)	WCRF/AICR (2017)
Consumption of whole grains		Per 90 g/day	0.83 (0.78-0.89)	WCRF/AICR (2017)
Consumption of dairy products		Per 400 g/day	0.87 (0.83-0.90)	WCRF/AICR (2017)
Milk intake		Per 200 g/day	0.94 (0.92-0.96)	WCRF/AICR (2017)
Calcium intake (dietary or	supplemented)	Per 300 mg/day	0.92 (0.89-0.95)	Keum et al (2014)
Physical activity (total level)		Low	1.00	WCRF/AICR (2017)
		High	0.81 (0.69-0.95)*	
Aspirin use		Never use	1.00	Yeet al (2013)
		Ever use	0.74 (0.64-0.83)	
		Per 325 mg/day	0.80 (0.74-0.88)	
		Per 7 times weekly	0.82 (0.78-0.87)	
		Per 10 years of use	0.82 (0.78-0.86)	
Hormone replacement therapy use		Never use	1.00	Green et al (2012)
		Ever use	0.84 (0.81-0.88)	
		Current use	0.77 (0.73-0.82)	
		Former use	0.89 (0.84-0.95)	
CI, confidence Interval; RR, relative risk. - A protective effect has been found for colon cancer (RR, 0.80; 95% CI, 0.72-0.88) but not for rectal cancer (RR, 1.04; 95% CI, 0.92-1.18).				

Source: IARC handbooks of cancer prevention. Colorectal cancer screening. Volume 17

2.1.3.1. Eating habits

Although not all epidemiological studies reach identical conclusions, it can be concluded that increased intake of fats (mainly of animal origin or saturated type) and red meat increases the risk of CRC OR=1.21 [1.13-1.29])[(73, 75)].

While fibre (vegetables and fruit), white meat (fish and poultry), calcium, vitamin D and folic acid are thought to be protective for both sexes. It is difficult to assess which foods and/or micronutrients play a role and what are the basic mechanisms that cause these tumours(74, 76, 77) (Table 5).

2.1.3.2. Overweight and obesity

Sedentary and overweight are two identified risk factors (74, 78, 79)).

For an increase in body mass index (BMI) of 5 kg/m^2 , the percentage increase in colorectal cancer risk was estimated to be 15%. In an obese person (BMI >30 kg/m^2), the increase in risk is 33% compared to a person with a BMI between 18 and 25 kg/m).[2]

Conversely, regular physical activity is a protective factor (80, 81) . The risk of developing colon cancer for men and women with high levels of physical activity is 18% and 20% lower, respectively, than for those with minimal physical activity(73) .

This correlation is not found in the case of rectal cancer(82) .

2.1.3.3. Tobacco

Studies agree that the risk is proportional to the number of cigarettes smoked and the number of years of smoking (83) .

The risk of CRC is higher the more years of smoking, the more cigarettes/day and the more packs/year: the OR is between 1.08 and 1.44 (meta-analysis including 36 prospective studies corresponding to 3 million subjects)(84) .

2.1.3.4. Alcohol

IARC has concluded that alcohol consumption is linked to colorectal cancer. A meta-analysis of 27 cohort and 34 case-control studies concluded that, compared to never drinkers, there is a significant increase in CRC risk for moderate (two to three drinks per day, RR 1.21, 95% CI 1.13-1.28) and heavy drinkers [>4 drinks per day, RR 1.52, 95% CI 1.27-1.81], but not light drinkers [>4 drinks per day, RR 1.52, 95% CI 1.27-1.81].4 drinks per day, RR 1.52, 95% CI 1.27-1.81), but not light drinkers [< 1 drink per day, RR 1.00, 95% CI 0.95-1.05](85) . The mechanisms involved are folate deficiency and the transformation of alcohol into acetaldehyde (a cancer-causing molecule) by the colonic microbiota(86) .

2.1.3.5. Other factors

- **Asbestos**

In 2005, a study showed that the occurrence of colon cancer is higher in workers exposed to asbestos(87) . According to the study, these workers had a 35% higher risk of developing colorectal cancer compared to a control group of non-asbestos exposed smokers.

In 2011, another case-control study confirmed the link between asbestos exposure and increased risk of colorectal cancer in the workplace(88) .

- **Diabetes and insulin resistance**

As the incidence of diabetes and obesity continues to rise in the developed world, **Tsilidis et al.** have demonstrated an increase in the relative risk of CRC incidence in subjects with diabetes (RR=1.27 [1.21; 1.34] (89) .

A recent meta-analysis of 29 prospective cohort studies (62,924 cases) in China reported a 27% higher risk of CRC associated with diabetes(90) . In a recent Chinese prospective study of 0.5 million participants with diabetes, the adjusted OR for CRC was 1.18 (95% CI: 1.04-1.33) (91).

- **Abdominal radiation**

Survivors of childhood malignancies who have received abdominal radiation have an increased risk of gastrointestinal neoplasms in adulthood, the majority of which are CRC. A clear radiation dose response effect on CRC risk has been noted with a 70% increase in risk for every 10 Gy increase in radiation dose. Exposure to an alkylating agent has an 8.8-fold increased risk of secondary CRC[(92)] . Men diagnosed with prostate cancer had an increased risk of subsequent CRC diagnosis (all CRC: OR = 1.14; 95% CI: 1.02-1.27; rectal cancer: OR = 1.36; 95% CI: 1.09-1.71). Treatment of prostate cancer with radiation was associated with an increased risk of rectal cancer (OR = 2.06; 95% CI: 1.42-2.99) compared with those not treated with radiation [(93, 94)].

2.2. Risk factors for gastric cancer

2.2.1. Non-modifiable factors

2.2.1.1. Individuals :

- **Age and gender :**

The risk of developing stomach cancer increases with age. It is highest after the age of 50. The average age at diagnosis in France is 74 for women and 71 for men **(INCa)**. In the USA, stomach cancer occurs most often in people over the age of 55. Most people diagnosed with stomach cancer are in their 60s and 70s[(95)] . Stomach cancer is more common in men than in women. The reasons for this difference are uncertain, but restrogen may have a protective effect[(1 3, 96, 97)] .

- **Blood type**

The relationship between stomach cancer and blood type A was first reported in 1953 by ***Aird et al.*** Numerous studies have shown that blood type A is associated with a higher risk of gastric cancer. An increase in pernicious anemia has also been observed in this group[(98)] .

- **Race/ethnicity**

Stomach cancer is more common in blacks, Hispanics and Asians than in whites[(99)] .

2.2.1.2. Personal history

- **Gastroesophageal reflux disease (GERD)**

Several studies have reported significant associations between GERD and gastric cancer of the cardia[(100)] . The incidence rate trends of reflux-related cardiac cancer and resophageal adenocarcinoma are very similar, suggesting that these two cancers share a similar etiology and pathophysiological process[(101)] .

- **Barrett's Esophagus**

This syndrome is clearly associated with distal and proximal gastric cancer. The fact of having undergone a partial gastrectomy (the risk increases by 10 to 15 after the operation, it would be multiplied by eight after 25 years).

- **Biermerian gastritis**

Due to Biermer's disease (which can, among other things, atrophy the glands of the gastric epithelium).

- Also mentioned are Menetrier's disease, gastric polyps (rare, especially if larger than 2 cm), gastric ulcer (not proven with certainty), gastric epithelial dysplasia and people treated for more than one year with gastric antisecretory drugs. **(Sources: World Cancer Research Fund**

International/American Institute for Cancer Research WCRF/AIRC 2007; HAS (Haute Autorite de la Sante), 2011; INCa, 2014; IARC; Canadian Cancer Society).

2.2.1.3. Genetic factors and antecedents

Genetic predisposition is considered to be a factor in the development of stomach cancer in 5-10% of cases.

- **Lynch syndrome (HNPCC)**

It is recognised as a risk factor for stomach cancer by the WCRF/AICR, INCa and HAS, although the risk is much lower than for CRC(102) .

Table 6: Cumulative risks of developing cancer in Lynch syndrome.

Risques cumulatifs avant 75 ans	Syndrome de Lynch	Population générale
Cancer colorectal	♀ : 24-52% ♂ : 28-75%	♀ : 3,5% ♂ : 4,6%
Cancer de l'endomètre	27-71%	1,5%
Cancer de l'estomac	2-13%	< 1%
Cancer de l'ovaire	3-13%	1,3%
Cancer des voies urinaires	1-12%	< 1%
Cancer de l'intestin grêle	4-7%	< 1%

Source: Swiss Medical Journal 2011; volume 7.1502-1506

- **Familial adenomatous polyposis (FAP)**

Most polyps develop on the lining of the colon and rectum, but they can, however, develop in the stomach and small intestine(103) .

- **Peutz-Jeghers syndrome.**
- **Juvenile Polyposis Syndrome** (The ARC Foundation, Canadian Society)
- **Hereditary diffuse gastric cancer (HDGC):**

According to the HAS, 1 to 3% of gastric cancers are hereditary. CGDH is characterised by autosomal dominant transmission of the mutated CDHI gene. Gastric cancer associated with CGDH usually appears before the age of 40.

The diagnosis is generally earlier than in sporadic forms (some patients under 18 years of age). Compared to sporadic forms, the 5-year survival prognosis (10%) is very poor **(INCa 2009; HAS, 2011).**

- **Family background**

A history of stomach cancer in the family is reported in 10-30% of cases (Agence nationale de securite sanitaire de l'alimentation, de l'environnement et du travail **ANSES, 2011; HAS, 2011).** Some studies have highlighted a higher risk of cancer in people who have a close family member (1er degree: parents, brothers/brothers) who has already been affected **(INCa, Canadian Society).** This risk remains fairly low but is the subject of a specific prevention approach(96) .

2.2.2. Modifiable and environmental factors

2.2.2.1. The role of infection (*Helicobacter pylon*)

Helicobacter *pylori* infection is the major causative factor in distal gastric cancer, accounting for 80% of cases, and has been the subject of much research(104,105) . The prevalence of this infection in the human population aged 50 years and over is higher in developing countries (74%) than in

developed countries (58%); these variations in prevalence are related to those of environmental factors[105].
Gastric cancer is the most common cancer associated with an infectious factor, coming before HPV cancers. This infection is acquired in childhood (probably through salivary or faecal route) and remains present for life if no treatment is carried out. It colonises the gastric mucosa and can lead to chronic gastritis, which in turn can promote the development of cancer. Approximately 1% of infected people will develop stomach cancer.

Helicobacter.pylori infection is one of the most important risk factors for stomach cancer, but it is one of the easiest to treat.

Approximately 5-10% of gastric carcinomas are associated with Epstein *Barr Virus* EBV[106]. Recent studies have shown that EBV and co-infection with *Helicobacter. pylori* increase the occurrence of gastric carcinoma[107].

2.2.2.2. Tobacco

Smoking is a definite risk factor for stomach cancer. There is sufficient epidemiological evidence to make such a conclusion. For habitual smokers, the risk of developing stomach cancer is increased by 53-57% compared to non-smokers **(IARC, 2012, Monograph Vol. 100 E).**

An estimated 11% of stomach cancers worldwide and 17% of cases in Europe are attributable to smoking[108]. A meta-analysis of 42 studies estimated that smokers had an approximately 1.53-fold increased risk of gastric cancer and that the risk was higher in men than in women[109]. A recent study showed that narguile and opium are risk factors for gastric cancer and precancerous lesions [110].

2.2.2.3. Alcohol

Alcohol consumption increases the risk of gastric cancer, but the effect of the amount of alcohol consumed and the risk of gastric cancer is controversial. Alcohol is known to irritate and erode the lining of the stomach, leading to gastritis, a precursor to stomach cancer[111].

2.2.2.4. Dietary factors

- **Salty food**

High dietary salt intake, including from salt-preserved foods (e.g. smoked or pickled with salt), greatly increases the risk of developing stomach cancer. The presence of salt makes *Helicobacter.pylori* infection more likely to occur and also appears to worsen the effect of the infection. In addition, salt damages the mucous membrane[108].
IARC (2012, Monograph 100 E) examined the consumption of dirty fish by the Chinese method and classified it as a definite carcinogen (Group 1) on the basis of sufficient evidence for nasopharyngeal cancer, and limited evidence for stomach cancer **(WCRF/AICR, 2007).** Japanese immigrants to the United States who assimilated and adopted Western foods had a significantly lower rate of gastric cancer than those who did not assimilate their diet[112].

- **Meat consumption**

Red meat fed on cereals is particularly high in saturated fats and low in protective fats such as omega-3, which contributes to its inflammatory processes and thus increases the risk of gastric cancer[112].

In terms of cooking methods for grilled or barbecued meat or fish, when these cooking methods are poorly controlled (excessive temperature and/or time, direct contact with the flame), there could be an increase in the levels of potentially cancer-causing compounds in the food (e.g. heterocyclic amines, acrylamide, hydrocarbons) **(INCa, 2009)**. However, the epidemiological evidence is considered to be limited by the WCRF/AICR[108].

- **Protective dietary factors**

Fruits and vegetables contain many antioxidants that prevent metabolic damage. Vitamin C, known as ascorbic acid, is a powerful antioxidant found in high concentrations in citrus fruits. Case-control studies have shown that high fruit and vegetable consumption reduces the risk of gastric cancer by 37%. Non-dietary antioxidant sources such as green tea, vitamin A, C and E supplements and selenium have had mixed results in preventing gastric cancer[108].

2.2.2.5. Obesite

A statistical meta-analysis from around the world found that people with excess body mass index (over 25 kg/m^2) have an odds ratio of 1.13 of developing cancer. The strength of the association increased with increasing BMI [108] **).**

2.2.2.6. Exposure to chemicals

Occupational exposure: IARC (1982, 2012 monograph Vol. 100F) retained exposure in rubber workers as a risk factor for stomach cancer. The IARC data retained **asbestos** exposure with limited evidence in humans for stomach cancer (Vol. 100C, 2012) and **inorganic lead compounds:** as probable carcinogens (Group 2A) (Sup 7, 87 2006) for stomach cancer. A recent meta-analysis of 13 observational studies showed that occupational exposure to talc is associated with an increased risk of stomach cancer[113].
Exposure to ionising radiation : Studies have shown that people exposed to radiation from nuclear accidents or fallout are also more likely to get stomach cancer. Some studies have reported that people treated with certain forms of radiation therapy have an increased risk of developing stomach cancer **(Canadian Society).**

2.3. Risk factors for HNV cancers

2.3.1. Non-modifiable risk factors :

2.3.1.1. Age and gender

Older people are more likely than younger people to develop biliary cancer. Most people diagnosed with biliary tract cancer are between 60 and 70 years old **(Cancer and the Environment)**.

2.3.1.2. Family history

A family history of biliary tract cancer seems to increase the risk of developing this disease, but the risk is low because it is a rare disease. Most biliary cancers are not found in people with a family history of the disease. **(American Cancer Society).**

2.3.1.3. Biliary tract disorders

- **Anomalies of the biliary-pancreatic junction or pancreaticobiliary junction: Bile duct cysts:**

Biliary cysts are rare congenital disorders characterized by cystic dilatation of the HBEV and/or intrahepatic bile ducts[114].

Biliary cysts are an established risk factor for CC. Type I (solitary, extrahepatic) and IV (extrahepatic and intrahepatic) biliary cysts have the highest incidence of CC[115]. The risk of malignancy decreases after complete cyst excision; however, these patients are still at increased risk of developing CC compared to the general population[116].

- **Biliary lithiasis (or gallstones)**

Symptomatic (chronic cholecystitis lesions are found in more than 75% of gallbladder cancers).

- **Primary sclerosing cholangitis :**

Primary sclerosing cholangitis is an autoimmune disease. It causes inflammation of the bile ducts (cholangitis), which leads to the formation of scar tissue (sclerosis).

- **Intravesicular polyps and calcifications of the gallbladder mucosa (porcelain gallbladder).**

2.3.1.4. Inflammatory bowel disease

Inflammatory bowel disease includes ulcerative colitis and Crohn's disease. People with these diseases have an increased risk of biliary tract cancer. A SEER-Medicare study showed a positive association of extrahepatic CC with Crohn's disease.

2.3.2. Modifiable risk factors

2.3.2.1. Infections

- **The hepatobiliary flukes *Opisthorchis viverrini (O. viverrini)* and *Clonorchis sinensis (C. sinensis)***

They are associated with the development of CC, particularly in South East Asia. Infection in humans occurs through ingestion of raw, marine or undercooked fish[117].

- **Chronic viral hepatitis and cirrhosis**

Hepatitis C virus (HCV), hepatitis B virus (HBV) and liver cirrhosis are potential risk factors for cholangiocarcinoma[118].

2.3.2.2. Other factors :

- **Obesity :**

Gallbladder cancer is one of the 10 cancer sites associated with excess weight, a modifiable nutritional factor, with a convincing level of evidence. The latest data from the 2015 WCRF/AICR update on gallbladder cancer reconfirms the importance of preventing overweight and obesity through a balanced and diversified diet and regular physical activity.

- **Alcohol :**

Some studies have found a link between alcohol consumption and an increased risk of bile duct cancer. The risk appears to be highest in heavy drinkers, people with alcoholic liver disease and people with primary sclerosing cholangitis.

- **Smoking :**

Some studies have found a link between smoking and an increased risk of bile duct cancer.

- **Diabetes :**

People with diabetes (type 1 or type 2) have an increased risk of biliary cancer. This increased risk is not high and the overall risk of biliary cancer in a person with diabetes is still low. However, the SEER-Medicare study showed a significant positive association between diabetes and BC.

2.4. Risk factors for pancreatic cancer

The risk factors for pancreatic cancer are either not well known or account for only a small proportion of pancreatic cancer.

2.4.1. Non-modifiable risk factors

2.4.1.1. Personal factors :

- **Age and gender :**

The risk of developing pancreatic cancer increases with age. Pancreatic cancer is not common before the age of 50. It occurs on average at the age of 69 in men and 74 in women **(Canadian Society).** It is twice as common in men (sex ratio 1.8).

- **ABO blood group**

More than 60 years ago, the role of ABO blood group in cancer biology was intensively studied by several researchers, and it is now widely recognized that ABO antigens are associated with the risk of developing several types of cancer, such as pancreatic[(119)] .

- **Chronic pancreatitis**

In recent decades, increasing evidence has defined chronic pancreatitis as a significant risk factor for pancreatic cancer[(120)] .

Chronic calcific pancreatitis is a risk factor for pancreatic cancer (relative risk of 1.8 to 2 at ten years).

Pancreatic adenocarcinoma is thought to occur in only 5% of patients with calcific chronic pancreatitis.

- **Pre-cancerous pancreatic lesions:**

These are mainly TIPMP (Intracanal mucinous and papillary tumours of the pancreas) and mucinous cystadenoma; among the cystic tumours of the pancreas, mucinous cystadenomas have an estimated 50% risk of degeneration.

2.4.1.2. Family and genetic factors :

Seven to ten percent of people with pancreatic cancer have a first-degree relative who was ill. Genetic variation or mutation plays an important role in increasing the risk of pancreatic cancer, the most commonly found being the *BRCA2* gene mutation, identified in 5-17% of familial pancreatic cancer cases[(121)] .

Pancreatic cancer is also associated with certain familial cancer syndromes such as hereditary non-polyposis colon cancer HNPCC (Lynch syndrome), familial multiple atypical melanoma syndrome, Peutz-Jeghers syndrome, hereditary breast and ovarian cancer, *Familial Athypical Multiple Mole Melanoma* **syndrome (FAMMM**), Familial Adenomatous Polyposis Li-Fraumeni Syndrome.

2.4.2. Modifiable risk factors :

2.4.2.1. Tobacco

The International Agency for Research on Cancer has confirmed that smoking is associated with pancreatic cancer. The risk of pancreatic cancer increases with the duration of smoking and the number of cigarettes smoked daily. The risk is almost twice as high in smokers as in non-smokers. In addition, a recent meta-analysis of 82 studies found that the relative risk of pancreatic cancer is 1.74 for former smokers and the risk persists for at least 10 years after quitting[(122)].

2.4.2.2. Alcohol

On the basis of numerous studies, the risk of pancreatic cancer is undoubtedly increased by high alcohol consumption (more than three drinks per day), whereas no association has been found with low to moderate alcohol consumption

[(123)]. However, low to moderate alcohol consumption was associated with an increased risk of pancreatic cancer in current smokers[(124)].

2.4.2.3. Obesite

Obesity is associated with an increased risk of several types of cancer, including pancreatic cancer[(125)]. Some studies have shown that obesity increases the incidence and mortality of pancreatic cancer. A study by **Li and Morris** showed that being overweight (body mass index (BMI): 25.0 - 29.9 kg/m^2) or obese (BMI > 30 kg/m^2) in early adulthood is associated with a higher risk of pancreatic cancer. Obesity in later life (30-79 years) is associated with poorer overall survival.

2.4.2.4. Dietary factors

Dietary factors have a 30-50% impact on pancreatic cancer, and there is evidence that some foods are associated with a higher risk, while others are even protective[(126)].
Consumption of red meat (especially when cooked at high temperatures), processed meats, cholesterol, fried foods and other foods containing nitrosamines may increase the risk of pancreatic cancer.

2.4.2.5. Diabetic sugar

About 80% of people with pancreatic cancer also have impaired glucose tolerance or diabetes. The association between these two diseases is clear but it is important to define the relationship. The majority of pancreatic cancer patients develop diabetes after the diagnosis of the tumour. But there is also a relevant association with type 2 diabetes with OR = 1.8[(127)].

2.4.2.6. Professional factors

The etiological fraction of pancreatic cancer due to occupational exposures (involving exposure to metallurgy and pesticides) in a population has been estimated at 12%.

- **X-rays and radiation**

Studies have shown a positive association between exposure to X-rays and radiation and pancreatic cancer **(Preston, 2007)**. However, there is no significant evidence of a dose-response relationship **(IARC, vol 100D, 2012)**.

- **Pesticides**

For pesticides, contradictory results have been obtained in agricultural populations. Only one study found positive associations between pesticide exposure and pancreatic cancer **(Bassil, 2007)**. But these results remain controversial and further studies are needed to validate them.

The Inserm collective expertise of June 2013 notes the limited experimental results available but stresses that particular attention should be paid to pesticides that may activate oestrogenic pathways at the pancreatic level **(Inserm, Collective expertise, 2013).**

- **Other sources of exposure**

A meta-analysis of occupational exposures and pancreatic cancer reported an increased risk with nickel exposure.

Few studies have found a link between cadmium and arsenic exposure and the risk of pancreatic cancer. Arsenic exposure has been associated with an increased risk of cancer **(IARC).**

Selenium, which is an essential trace element, has been inversely associated with several cancers, including pancreatic cancer[(128)] . Selenium also appears to act as an antagonist to arsenic, cadmium and lead, reducing the oxidative stress caused by exposure to these elements.

2.5. Risk factors for liver cancer

The risk of getting liver cancer increases with age. It affects men more than women. Liver cancer is more common in countries with high rates of hepatitis B and hepatitis C infection.

The main risk factors are those that cause cirrhosis, but there are also others[(129)] .

2.5.1. **Hereditary liver diseases** (hereditary Hemochromatosis)

Hereditary hemochromatosis is an autosomal recessive hereditary disorder. It is characterised by increased dietary iron absorption resulting in progressive deposition of iron in several organs, but particularly in the liver. The disorder is the result of mutations in a number of genes involved in iron absorption[(130)] . The incidence of liver cancer in patients with hemochromatosis is 8% to 10% in most surveys, with the tumour accounting for up to 45% of deaths. Cirrhosis is present in almost all patients who develop the tumour[(131)] .

2.5.2. Non-alcoholic fatty liver disease

It is a condition similar to alcoholic fatty liver disease, but it causes fat to accumulate in the liver (fatty liver disease) by a different mechanism. It is thought to be an autoimmune disease (in which the body makes antibodies against itself) and may have a genetic component[(132)] .
In France, according to the **Societe Nationale Fran^aise de Gastroenterologie**, in 20% of cases, this steatosis causes liver inflammation which can lead to cirrhosis and liver cancer. The prevalence of hepatic steatosis is 18.2%. Projections estimate that this number will more than double by 2030, and that complications of cirrhosis and hepatocellular carcinoma related to non-alcoholic fatty liver disease will triple by then.

2.5.3. Chronic hepatitis B virus (HBV) or hepatitis C virus (HCV) infections

HBV or HCV infection is considered chronic when the hepatitis virus remains present in the blood for more than six months and interferes with liver function. Worldwide, hepatitis B infection is responsible for 50% of all cases of liver cancer, and hepatitis C infection for 25% of cases. Chronic hepatitis B infection increases the risk of developing liver cancer 100-fold and chronic hepatitis C infection increases the risk 17-fold. Up to 85% of people infected with hepatitis C develop a chronic infection, of which 30% will progress to cirrhosis, and each year 1-2% of these develop liver cancer. Co-infection with HBV, i.e. infection with both types of virus occurring at the same time, greatly increases this risk [(133)].

2.5.4. Other factors :

- **Alcohol**

Long-term alcohol abuse can lead to cirrhosis and liver cancer. In countries where HBV infection is low, alcohol is the main cause of liver cancer. Drinking alcohol while suffering from hepatitis multiplies the risk (134)

A meta-analysis showed a dose-response relationship between alcohol consumption and HCC with relative risks of 1.19 (95% CI: 1.12-1.27), 1.40 (95% CI: 1.25-1.56) and 1.81 (95% CI: 1.50-2.19) with alcohol intakes of 25, 50 and 100 g per day, respectively[(135)] . Chronic alcohol consumption over at least 10 years significantly increases the risk of HCC development in patients chronically infected with HCV or HBV, compared to patients with a viral infection who do not drink too much alcohol. In addition, the tumour may occur earlier in these patients[(134)] .

- **Aflatoxin :**

Aflatoxin is a mycotoxin produced by Aspergillus flavus and an apparent fungus that contaminates stored foods such as rice, maize, soybeans and peanuts. In some parts of the world, particularly in Asia and Africa, these are the main risk factors for HCC.

- **Obesite**

A recent meta-analysis showed that the relative risk of HCC was 1.17 (95% CI: 1.02 to 1.34) in overweight people and 1.89 (95% CI: 1.51-2.36) in obese people (BMI> 30 kg/m2)[(136)] .

- **Smoking**

A relatively small number of studies have addressed smoking as a cause of liver cancer. These studies have shown increased odds ratios for tumour development in smokers. **IARC** considers smoking to be a risk factor, and most authorities agree with this conclusion.

- **Diabetes**

It seems that people with diabetes are at greater risk of developing liver cancer. Studies have shown that people with diabetes who develop liver cancer may have other risk factors such as excessive alcohol consumption, hepatitis infection or both. Many people with diabetes also tend to be overweight or obese, which can also increase their risk of liver cancer **(Canadian Society).**

- **Exposure to toxic agents:**

Anabolic steroids are hormones taken by some athletes to increase strength and muscle mass. Long-term use of these substances increases the risk of hepatocellular adenoma, a benign liver tumour that can become malignant and develop into HCC[(133)] .

2.6. Risk factors for resophageal cancer

Adenocarcinoma and squamous cell carcinoma have different risk factors. Gastro-resophageal reflux disease and obesity are risk factors for developing adenocarcinoma on Barett's resophagus, whereas squamous cell carcinoma is related to alcohol and tobacco abuse, consumption of hot drinks and achalasia. Squamous cell cancer is often associated with ENT cancers.

2.6.1. Individual and genetic risk factors

Age. People aged 45 to 70 years have the highest risk of resophageal cancer.

Gender and race: Squamous cell carcinoma is the most common histological type in black individuals and white women, while adenocarcinoma is predominant in white men (P <0.001)[(137)] . Men are 3 to 4 times more likely than women to develop resophageal cancer.

Genetics: There are genetically based conditions, such as tylosis, an autosomal dominant disease, which are clearly linked to the development of esophageal squamous cell carcinoma. Familial aggregation in the population with a high incidence of resophageal carcinoma, such as in the northern regions of China, has also been reported[(138)] .

2.6.2. Medical history

- **Gastro-resophageal reflux disease and Barrett's resophagus :**

Barrett's resophagus is a pre-malignant lesion that develops in 6% to 14% of GERD patients and of which approximately 0.5% to 1% will develop adenocarcinoma (139).

In a study from Spain, the incidence of adenocarcinoma during follow-up of patients with Barrett's resophagus was 0.48% per year (95% CI: 0.006% - 2.62%), with an incidence of 1 per 210 patient-years[(140)] .

- **Certain pathologies:**

Achalasia increases the risk of developing squamous cell carcinoma. Achalasia is a condition in which the muscle that closes the lower end of the esophagus cannot relax properly. Swallowed food and fluids therefore tend to accumulate in the resophagus, which expands at its lower end.

Other rare diseases such as diffuse palmoplantar keratoderma and Plummer-Vinson syndrome also increase the risk of squamous cell carcinoma of the resophagus[(141)] .

2.6.3. Habits

- **Smoking :**

Smoking or chewing tobacco is one of the main risk factors for developing resophageal squamous cell carcinoma. Smokers are twice as likely to develop this disease as non-smokers[(142)] . The risk increases with the total duration of smoking and the number of cigarettes smoked per day[(141)] .

- **Obesity :**

Obesity is a major and consistent risk factor for the development of resophageal adenocarcinoma. The OR for the development of adenocarcinoma is 1.52 (95% CI: 1.33-1.74, *P* <0.0001) for those with a BMI in the 25-30 range compared with those of normal weight. A high BMI (>25) is associated with an increased risk of resophageal adenocarcinoma (men, OR = 2.2; 95% CI: 1.7-2.7; women, OR = 2.0; 95% CI: 1.4-2.9) (143).

- **Alcohol consumption:**

The risk of developing squamous cell carcinoma is related to the amount of alcohol consumed. The relative risk increases with the amount of alcohol consumed, ranging from 1.8 to 7.4 depending on the weekly volume[(142)] . The combination of alcohol consumption and smoking further increases the risk.

- **Dietary factors**

Global dietary deficiencies have been blamed in high-risk areas of Iran or China where tobacco and alcohol play virtually no role in the etiology of the disease. In addition to poverty and monotony of diet, other exogenous factors have been suggested.

Tea, mate and coffee have been extensively studied as potential risk factors associated with resophageal carcinoma and its geographical distribution, particularly in South American regions. There is little evidence of a cancerogenic relationship across its components, except for mate, which is related to both quantity consumed and temperature[(142)] . Low consumption of fresh fruit and vegetables.

- **Consumption of betel quid:**

Betel quid is a mixture of plants consumed in many South Asian cultures. The leaves of the betel plant have a stimulating effect, but also slightly increase the risk of cancer of the esophagus[(142)] .

2.7. Risk factors for small bowel cancer

2.7.1. Non-modifiable risk factors

- **Age and gender**

The risk of developing bowel cancer increases with age. Most people who are diagnosed are around 60 years old. Adenocarcinoma of the grafted bowel affects men slightly more than women.

In the United States, the median age for diagnosis of graft bowel cancer is 66 years(144) . After about 40 years of age, the risk of graft bowel cancer begins to increase and does not appear to stabilise until about age 90.

- **Hereditary mutations**
- **Familial adenomatous polyposis (FAP)**: The grafted bowel is the second most common site of adenocarcinoma in FAP (duodenum). The risk of adenocarcinoma of the grafted bowel in people with FAP is 330 times higher than in the general population(145) .
- **Lynch syndrome**

The lifetime risk of adenocarcinoma of the grafted bowel in patients with Lynch syndrome remains low, around 1% according to a French registry(146) .

- **Peutz-Jeghers syndrome**
- **Multiple endocrine neoplasia syndrome type 1**
- **Neurofibromatosis type 1.**

- **Inflammatory bowel disease**

Inflammatory bowel disease is most often caused by Crohn's disease or ulcerative colitis. Crohn's disease is a hereditary autoimmune disease that causes inflammation in the intestine, most commonly affecting the ileum(147) .

- **Celia disease**

A French prospective study found that predisposing or hereditary diseases were involved in 20% of cases: 8.6% had Crohn's disease, 3% had PAF, 3% had Lynch syndrome, 1.5% had celiac disease. Of the metastatic patients, 14.7% had Crohn's disease and 5.9% had Lynch syndrome(148) .

History of colorectal and other cancers (ovarian, stomach and pancreas).

2.7.2. Modifiable risk factors

- **Food**

Diets high in animal fat and animal protein have been associated with a higher risk of cancer of the small intestine. One study specifically challenged the cancer-causing effects of meat, but found an association between cancer of the small intestine and saturated fats, found in large quantities in meat (149).

- **Alcohol**

Several studies have found a slight positive association between alcohol and adenocarcinoma of the grafted bowel, while several others have not due to the rarity of the disease(150) .

- **Tobacco**

Several studies have shown that smoking increases the risk of graft bowel cancer(151) .

- **Obesite**

Many studies have investigated a correlation between obesity and graft bowel cancer, with mixed results. One study found a relative risk of 1.5 in people diagnosed as obese(151) .

- **Occupational hazards**

Several studies have found numerous occupations that were associated with an increased risk of cancer of the small intestine. One study found a high risk among Australian nuclear workers, despite the fact that radiation exposure for these workers is strictly regulated. Other occupations, involved in a separate study, included shoemakers, ironworkers, painters and other construction workers(152) .

CHAPTER 3

PREVENTION OF DIGESTIVE CANCERS

According to WHO, prevention aims at the early detection of diseases, with the aim of discovering them at an early stage when they can be treated **(Gaye, 2011)**

In the case of cancer, screening consists of detecting it at its earliest stage (cure 9 times out of 10 at stage I) or detecting possible precancerous lesions before the person feels the symptoms. Screening can be an individual, spontaneous or private request. But it can also be done in the context of a collective public health action **(Parente, 2010)**.

3.1. Primary prevention

Primary prevention strategies are classically based on the prevention of modifiable risk factors.

Experimental and epidemiological studies suggest the role of a number of modifiable exogenous factors that are common to the different digestive cancers, the main ones being dietary habits, alcohol consumption, smoking and sedentariness (**see Chapter 2**).
The international collective expertise carried out by the WCRF and the AICR in 2007 allowed the relationship between nutritional factors and cancer risk to be qualified as "convincing", "probable", "limited but suggestive", "unlikely", taking into account the diversity of populations and their exposure to these nutritional factors.

Controlling modifiable risk factors (smoking, alcohol consumption) and modifying lifestyle habits (increasing physical activity or the proportion of fibre in the diet) are proven or likely to be effective in preventing digestive cancers.

Reducing alcohol consumption and stopping smoking

- **Alcohol :**

Abstainers should not be encouraged to drink regularly, even in moderation, as regular alcohol consumption is a risk for colorectal cancer.
If alcohol is consumed, in order to reduce the risk of cancer, it is advisable to limit consumption as much as possible, both in terms of quantity and frequency of consumption.

- **Tobacco:**

Smokers should be encouraged to stop smoking as soon as possible or at least to reduce their consumption considerably.

- **Reduction in the consumption of meat and sausages**

To prevent the risk of cancer, the consumption of red meat should be limited to less than 500g per week. To complete the protein intake, it is advisable to alternate with white meat, fish, eggs and legumes.

It is also advisable to limit the consumption of cold meats, especially very fatty and/or very dirty ones.

- **Increase in dietary fibre intake**

A diet rich in fibre (wholegrain cereals, fruit, vegetables, pulses) is associated with a lower risk of developing colorectal cancer (probable level of evidence).

- **Consumption of dairy products**

According to meta-analyses carried out by the WCRF/AICR in 2007, milk consumption is likely to be associated with a reduced risk of colorectal cancer (however, a calcium-rich diet in excess of 2 times the recommended intake would increase the risk of prostate cancer).

- **Increased physical activity**

Physical activity is associated with a decreased risk of colorectal cancer, with an estimated percentage decrease in risk for physically active individuals compared to non-active individuals ranging from 18% to 29% for moderate to regular physical activity and 50% for those with intense physical activity.

-The main mechanisms that could explain the beneficial effect of physical activity on the risk of cancer would be linked to its effects on the circulating levels of various hormones and growth factors: reduction, among others, of the plasma levels of insulin and IGF-1, which are increased by overweight and obesity and which promote cell proliferation.

Physical activity may also specifically reduce the risk of colon cancer by accelerating bowel movements, thereby reducing the exposure time of the digestive mucosa to food-borne cancerogens.

- **Weight standardisation**

To reduce the risk of cancer associated with excess weight, it is recommended to maintain a normal weight (BMI between 18.5 and 25 kg/m).[2]

To prevent overweight and obesity, it is recommended to practise regular physical activity, to limit the consumption of energy-dense foods and to favour energy-dense foods (fruits and vegetables).

Regular weight monitoring should be advised (weigh yourself once a month).

- **Infections**

It is hoped that eradication of *Helicobacter pylori* infection by antibiotic therapy will reduce the incidence of gastric cancer. A randomised trial of antibiotic therapy has been conducted in a cohort of patients with resectable gastric cancer, with the aim of preventing second primary cancers[(153)] .

Vaccination against hepatitis B and prevention of hepatitis C.

- **Chemoprophylaxis**
- **Aspirin:** Several agents (notably NSAIDs) have been shown to have modest to moderate chemopreventive effects in populations at intermediate and high risk of CRC[(154)] . A meta-analysis showed that regular aspirin use is associated with a reduced risk of colorectal cancer [RR = 0.73, 95% CI = 0.69-0.78], squamous cell carcinoma of the resophagus (RR = 0.67, 95% CI = 0.57-0.79), adenocarcinoma of the resophagus and gastric cardia (RR = 0.61, 95% CI = 0.49-0.77), gastric cancer (RR = 0.64, 95% CI = 0.51-0.82), biliary tract cancer (RR = 0.62, 95% CI = 0.44-0.86) and pancreatic cancer (RR = 0.78, 95% CI = 0.68-0.89) [(155)].
- **Sulindac plus DFMO or erlotinib** - Chemoprophylaxis with the combination of difluoromethylornithine (DFMO) and sulindac (an NSAID drug) has been evaluated in a randomised controlled trial 5[(16)] .

3.2. Secondary prevention: screening ++.

3.2.1. Colorectal cancer screening

Colorectal cancer screening is based primarily on the ability to identify early stage cancers in the colon and rectum and the presence of adenomatous polyps, which are truly precarious conditions.

Detection of the disease at an early stage that has not yet metastasised can reduce not only mortality but also incidence[157] . The occurrence of cancer can be effectively prevented by the detection and removal of colorectal adenomas, which are responsible for more than 95% of cancers.

Colorectal cancer screening involves two distinct procedures:

> A community-based organised screening programme is offered as part of a national campaign of age-specific screening (50-74 years) using a faecal occult blood test (Hemoccult II test). In this programme, the screening test is used to sort out men or women with fecal occult blood in an apparently healthy target population who are likely to have colorectal cancer.
> An opportunistic individual screening, during a consultation, patients are invited to be screened, if the consulting physician has identified in these people :
S personal or family history of excess risk of colorectal cancer;
S of functional signs necessitating the implementation of the individual screening procedure by colonoscopy.

Organised screening for people at moderate risk based on an immunological test for occult blood in the stool, and in case of a positive result, a colonoscopy.

Individualised screening for people at high and very high risk who are initially referred for colonoscopy.

3.2.1.1. Screening in medium risk groups

People at average risk **(see Chapter 2)** are candidates for general screening for fecal occult bleeding. This screening concerns men and women over 50 years of age in the general population who are neither at high nor very high risk[158] .

Stool occult blood testing is a suitable method for early stage detection. There are two types of tests using this method: gaiac tests and immunological tests[159] .

- **Gaiac tests** (Hemoccult)

The Gaiac test consists of collecting two small stool fragments from three consecutive stools. The stool fragments must be placed on the Gaiac impregnated reagent paper. Once returned to the reading centre, a drop of oxygenated water is deposited, in case of a positive result a blue coloration appears. Colonoscopies performed in case of a positive Hemoccult find an adenoma and/or cancer in 42% of cases[158] .

- **Immunological tests**

The principle of immunochemical tests is based on the specific detection of human hemoglobin using monoclonal or polyclonal antibodies recognising the globin part of hemoglobin. These tests are more specific than tests based on the demonstration of pseudoperoxidase activity. Their sensitivity measured in the laboratory (from a colonic blood loss of 0.25 ml per day) is superior to that of the gaiac tests (from a colonic blood loss of 0.5 ml per day).

Finally, as globin is rapidly digested in the stomach and the grafted intestine, immunological tests are in principle more specific than guaiac tests[159] .

3.2.1.2. Screening in high risk groups

This population includes people with a family history of CRC and those with chronic inflammatory bowel disease, Crohn's disease or ulcerative colitis **(Pariente ,2014).**

3.2.1.3. Screening in high risk groups

- **Familial adenomatous polyposis**

The responsible mutation can be identified in 90% of affected subjects, allowing a family-oriented screening: genetic diagnosis around 10-12 years of age looking for the presence of the identified mutation in the affected parent, then annual recto-sigmoido-scopy in subjects carrying the mutation. **(Pariente ,2014).**

- **Hereditary non-polyposis colon cancer syndrome** (HNPCC)

The International Consortium on HNPCC sets out the so-called Amsterdam criteria for clinical definition of the syndrome:

- Three relatives with histologically proven CRC, one of whom must be first-degree related to the other two;
- At least two successive generations reached;
- One of the cancers diagnosed before the age of 50;
- Exclusion of familial rectocolic polyposis.

According to studies in unselected populations, 2-3% of colorectal cancers occur in the context of Lynch syndrome **(Hemminki, 2001, Katballe, 2002).**

In affected individuals, monitoring is recommended:

- a total colonoscopy every two years from the age of 25 or five years before the age at which the earliest case in the family was diagnosed.
- an annual gynecological examination from the age of 30 with endovaginal ultrasound and Pap smear.
- there is no consensus on the surveillance of other digestive or urinary tract cancers due to their lower frequency[(160)] .

- Polyposis linked to the *MUTYH* gene

Polyposis related to a mutation in the *MUTYH* gene is of more recent knowledge. The particularity of this predisposition is its recessive transmission, i.e. affected subjects have received a mutated allele from each of their parents and a quarter of the children will be affected. It is important to consider this when there is a polyposis without PAF in the family (especially in the attenuated forms). Their descendants will not be affected unless the spouse also carries a *MUTYH* mutation. As a precaution, a genetic test can be proposed to children[(159)] .

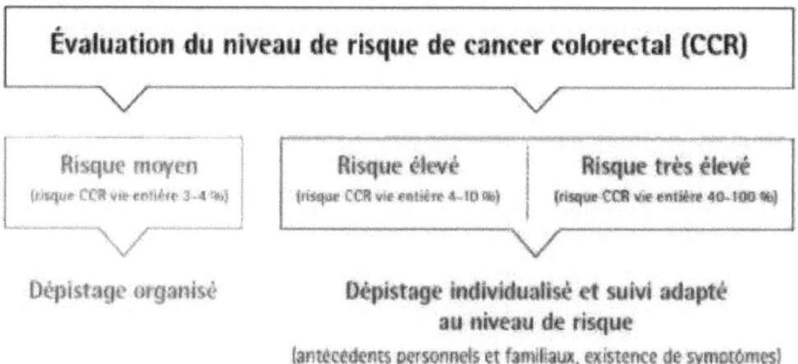

Colorectal cancer screening. HAS [60]

In Algeria, a colorectal cancer screening campaign in the Wilaya of Bejaia started in 2017, targeting women and men aged 50 to 70. However, the objective formulated in terms of participation rate was not reached. In addition to the low screening coverage, patients referred for colonoscopy found it difficult to benefit from this examination, in addition to a problem with the quality assurance of this screening.

3.2.2. Individual screening for some digestive cancers

3.2.2.1. Stomach cancer

Gastric cancer screening usually involves contrast radiography and endoscopy[161] . Other non-invasive methods used are serum pepsinogen levels, *Helicobacter. pylori* serology and trefoil serum factor 3, although their use has been controversial. Further studies are needed to define the role of these non-invasive methods of gastric cancer screening.

Endoscopy allows direct visual examination of the gastric mucosa and enables biopsy and histological evaluation. In Japan, gastric cancer screening is performed annually for all residents over the age of 40[162] . Similarly, in Korea, endoscopy is recommended every two years for people aged 40 and over[161] .

> Family risk of stomach cancer

- Risk of stomach cancer increases in first-degree relatives of a patient with stomach cancer.
- Frequency of *Helicobacter. pylori* infection and precancerous gastric mucosal lesions (atrophy, intestinal metaplasia and dysplasia) in first degree relatives.
- This risk justifies a specific prevention approach:

If under 40 years of age: test for Helicobacter *pylori* by breath test or serology.
After 10 years: endoscopic exploration of the stomach for *Helicobacter. pylori* and precancerous lesions.

> Subjects at risk of cancer

- Countries with a high incidence of gastric cancer: mass screening for *Helicobacter.pylori* infection, systematic preventive treatment of infection early in life.
- Countries with lower incidence: routine screening for infection not recommended; need to select patients at high risk of stomach cancer for treatment of infection.
- Main categories of patients at risk:
- Persons related to a patient who has had stomach cancer in the 1er degree.
- Patients who have had a partial gastrectomy for superficial cancer (mucosectomy or submucosal dissection).

- Patients with precancerous lesions of the stomach: severe pangastritis or predominantly body stomach, severe atrophy and/or extensive intestinal metaplasia, dysplasia, Biermer's disease, Menetrier's disease.
- Patients treated with PPI for more than one year.
- Subjects from countries with a high incidence of cancer (Asian or South American countries).
- Subjects with a predisposition syndrome for digestive cancers (HNPCC/Lynch).

- **Endoscopic investigation of individuals at risk of gastric cancer**
- Endoscopy as a first-line treatment in at-risk subjects over 40 years of age.
- Careful examination of the gastric mucosa. Surface staining and virtual chromoscopy facilitate the detection of foci of intestinal metaplasia.
- Systematically perform at least 5 gastric biopsies, even in the absence of obvious lesions, 2 of which are of the body of the stomach.
- Cancer risk stratification by histological scores (OLGA and OLGIM) according to severity and topography of chronic atrophic gastritis and intestinal metaplasia lesions.

3.2.2.2. Pancreatic cancer

Screening of large groups in the general population is not currently considered effective in detecting early stage disease, although newer techniques and screening of narrowly targeted groups (particularly those with a family history) are being evaluated 3, [16164]**These** include the pancreatic cancer blood markers CA19-9, CA-50, SPAN-1, DUPAN-2, cell surface associated mucins (CSAM), carcinoembryonic antigen and heat shock proteins. However, these tests have not yet been well studied. Furthermore, screening efforts have so far focused on the detection of precancerous lesions.

Screening for precancerous lesions and familial forms

- **Pre-cancerous lesions**

They include intraepithelial neoplasia, TIPMP and mucinous cystadenoma[165] . Radiological signs of concern have been defined to guide the operative indications for these lesions[166] . The following indications are in favour of resection:

For TIPMP :

- relative indications: Wirsung duct diameter between 5 and 9.9 mm or (secondary duct > 40 mm, growth > 5 mm/year, CA19.9 >37 U/mL in the absence of icterus, recent onset diabetes, acute pancreatitis, and wall nodule < 5 mm in diameter.
- absolute indications: icterus, mural nodule > 5 mm taking contrast, solid mass or diameter of the Wirsung canal > 10 mm, positive cytology (cancer or high grade dysplasia)

For mucinous cystadenomas: diameter > 40 mm, or contrast-enhancing nodule.

For non-operated patients, monitoring by MRI and/or EE is recommended every 6 months for the first year, then annually[166] .

- **Genetic forms**

- Genetic susceptibility would explain about 5%-10% of pancreatic adenocarcinomas **(de**

Mestier, Vedie, Salfati, Rebours, & Hammel, 2017; Ryan, Hong, & Bardeesy, 2014).

- Familial pancreatic cancers are defined by the occurrence of pancreatic adenocarcinoma in at least 2 first-degree relatives, or in the presence of at least 3 cases from the same branch regardless of degree of relationship and age of occurrence.

- The risk of developing PA increases with the number of affected relatives **(Canto et al. 2013; de Mestier et al. 2016; de Mestier et al. 2017).**

- Hereditary predisposing conditions and syndromes are associated with an increased risk of developing pancreatic adenocarcinoma.

- **Screening**

- The aim of pancreatic adenocarcinoma screening is to detect precancerous lesions that are amenable to early curative surgical management and therefore only in subjects eligible for pancreatic surgery.

- It applies to individuals with a cumulative theoretical lifetime risk of pancreatic adenocarcinoma >5% or an estimated relative risk >5: having > 2 relatives with pancreatic adenocarcinoma including > 1 in the first degree; carriers of a germline predisposition gene mutation and having > 2 relatives with pancreatic adenocarcinoma or > 1 in the first degree; any patient with Peutz-Jeghers syndrome, regardless of family history.

After discussion of the potential benefits and risks of such screening. Screening modalities should be based on non-irradiating examinations (MRI).

3.3. Tertiary prevention

Tertiary prevention is used in the specific treatment of diseases or the prevention of complications associated with the disease, is often used to treat a type of cancer and metastases, or is used to treat patients at risk of developing a secondary primary cancer. The goal of tertiary prevention in cancer patients is to reduce morbidity and mortality with optimal treatment. Both primary and secondary prevention practices are recommended in developing and less developed countries because of the greater economic burden of tertiary prevention[(167)].

WHO (2002) describes cancer diagnosis as the first step in cancer management. It involves a combination of a clinical examination and a series of additional tests, such as endoscopy, imaging, histopathology, cytology and laboratory studies. Diagnostic tests are also important in the assessment of disease spread. Staging of cancer is necessary to determine treatment options and assessment of the likely prognosis. The treatment of cancer is complex, involving a range of therapies that include surgery, radiotherapy, chemotherapy or hormonal therapy or their combination. The aim of treatment is to cure people with cancer, or to prolong and improve the quality of life of people with cancer **(WHO, 2002).**

Tertiary prevention or surveillance in patients who have already had polyps or colorectal cancer aims to avoid the consequences of the development of these lesions. This group of patients should therefore be monitored colonoscopically for new polyps or recurrence of cancer as early as possible.

- **Supportive Care and Rehabilitation**

The impact of cancer on patients goes beyond the physical; the disease also has psychological, social, economic, sexual and spiritual consequences. Coping with the disease and its treatment involves a range of issues that impact on people with cancer and their families. Supportive care and rehabilitation involves the provision of necessary services, as determined by the people affected by cancer or those living with them, to meet their physical, social, emotional, nutritional, information, psychological, sexual, spiritual and practical needs. It is an approach that improves the quality of life of patients and their families in the face of problems associated with terminal illness, through the prevention and relief of suffering through early identification and proper assessment and treatment of pain and other physical, psychosocial and spiritual problems" (WHO 2002). Internationally, it is recognised that supportive and rehabilitative care is desirable at every stage along the continuum of care.

- **Role of physical activity**

Regular exercise has a well-known protective effect on the risk of certain cancers, notably colon, breast and endometrial cancer. However, the benefits of exercise after cancer diagnosis are less well known to patients and carers. In cancer patients, adapted physical activity, i.e. exercise that Taking into account the particularities of the individual, his or her disease and treatment, this practice is effective in reducing fatigue and improving quality of life; it could even positively influence patient survival. Adapted physical activity is currently being developed as a promising new therapeutic intervention modality in the field of supportive care and tertiary prevention in cancer[(168)] .

CHAPTER 4

ALGERIAN STRATEGY FOR THE FIGHT AGAINST CANCER

4.1. National Cancer Plan 2018 - 2019 (patient-centred strategic vision)

The main objective of this plan is to reduce cancer mortality and morbidity. It represents, in fact, an essential strategic axis which is the only one capable of demonstrating the efficiency of a health system.

This policy is based on three principles:

- Improving the fluidity of the patient journey,
- strengthening prevention and screening
- the development of effective therapeutic methods in which palliative care will find a more significant place.

STRATEGIC AREA 1 Improving prevention against risk factors Focus: Tobacco control

OBJECTIVE 1 Reduce tobacco use in the entire population and particularly among children, adolescents and young people

OBJECTIVE 2 Strengthen protection from exposure to tobacco smoke

OBJECTIVE 3 Creating supportive environments to reduce tobacco demand

OBJECTIVE 4 To provide smoking cessation support

OBJECTIVE 5 To create a monitoring system for smoking and its consequences

16 actions and 37 measures

STRATEGIC AXIS 2	Improving screening for certain cancers Focus: Breast cancer screening

OBJECTIVE 1 Organise breast cancer screening. **3 actions, 19 measures**.

STRATEGIC AXIS 3	Improving cancer diagnosis Focus: Anatomo CytoPathology

OBJECTIVE 1 To improve the services offered by CPA laboratories

OBJECTIVE 2 Improve medical imaging services

OBJECTIVE 3 Strengthen nuclear medicine services.

OBJECTIVE 4 Strengthen Biology services.

6 actions and 29 measures

STRATEGIC AREA 4 Revitalising treatment Focus: Interdisciplinarity

OBJECTIVE 1 Improving patient care: **10 actions and 43 measures**

STRATEGIC AXIS 5 Organising patient orientation, support and follow-up

Focus: Cancer patient support and referral units

OBJECTIVE 1 To provide psychological support for patients and their families
OBJECTIVE 2 Reduce barriers to access to cancer diagnosis and treatment centres **04 actions, 22 measures.**

STRATEGIC AREA 6 Developing the information system and communication on cancer

Focus: Cancer registries

OBJECTIVE 1 To improve epidemiological surveillance of cancers by establishing coordination of cancer registries
OBJECTIVE 2 Improve [information and communication on cancer
7 actions, 32 measures

STRATEGIC AREA 7 Strengthen cancer education and research

Focus: Introduction to new professions and cross-disciplinary research

OBJECTIVE 1 Optimise the training of all actors in the cancer care chain
OBJECTIVE 2 To develop cancer research
11 actions and 50 measures.

STRATEGIC AREA 8 Strengthening the capacity to fund cancer care

Focus: Optimising and rationalising available financial resources

OBJECTIVE 1 Optimise and rationalise the financial resources available
OBJECTIVE 2 Budgeting for prevention, training and research programmes
03 actions and 07 measures.

4.2. National multisectoral strategic plan for integrated control of risk factors for non-communicable diseases 2015 - 2019

Acting exclusively on risk factors does not allow sufficient involvement of all the actors concerned by the different problems targeted by this plan. It must be complemented by an approach by living environment or by age groups:

The educational community appears to be an essential partner in the promotion of health and the prevention of NCDs in future adults.

The period of secondary and higher education is a key moment in a young person's life.

The school medical services and the Preventive Medicine Units (UMP) play a crucial role through systematic medical visits in educational and university establishments.

Occupational health professionals play a preventive role through the detection of occupational diseases, as well as the monitoring of the health status and the psychological, mental and physical abilities of workers.

- The measures of the Plan are to be considered as **expected results**:

Measures relating to the development of living environments and infrastructure.
Measures relating to the development of health and health promotion services.
Measures relating to the accessibility of infrastructure as well as health, health promotion and social support services.
Measures relating to the mobilisation of political actors and institutional leaders.
Measures to support professionals and strengthen their outreach to the population.

OBJECTIVE

Develop coordinated and intersectoral action to address risk factors and their determinants and strengthen the prevention of non-communicable diseases

To achieve this objective, the Plan is divided into 4 strategic axes:

Axis 1. Promotion of healthy eating
Axis 2. Promotion of physical activity, sport and active mobility Axis 3. Tobacco control
Axis 4. Coordination framework

STRATEGIC AXIS 1 - PROMOTION OF HEALTHY EATING

Objective 1 Promote appropriate nutrition during pregnancy and exclusive breastfeeding up to 6 months: **3 actions and 10 measures**
Objective 2 To promote healthy eating among children, young people and adolescents in educational establishments, schools and preschools: **4 actions and 20 measures**
Objective 3 To promote healthy eating among the general population: **3 actions and 5 measures**
Objective 4 Reduce the daily consumption of: salt, sugar, fat in the general population: **2 actions and 6 measures**
Objective 5 Prevent obesity in the general population: 2 actions and 9 measures

STRATEGIC AXIS 2 - PROMOTION OF PHYSICAL ACTIVITY, SPORT AND ACTIVE MOBILITY

Objective 1 Promote the practice of physical activity and sport: **3 actions and 17 measures**
Objective 2 Promote active mobility: **3 actions and 10 measures**

STRATEGIC AXIS 3 - TOBACCO CONTROL

Objective 1 To strengthen tobacco control legislation and regulation in line with the provisions of the FCTC: **1 action and 6 measures**
Objective 2 Creating a supportive environment to reduce smoking: **4 actions and 11 measures**
Objective 3 To provide smoking cessation support: **2 actions and 8 measures**
Objective 4 To establish a comprehensive and permanent tobacco monitoring system: **2 actions and 6 measures**

STRATEGIC AXIS 4 - COORDINATION FRAMEWORK

Objective 1 Institutionalise a multi-sectoral coordination framework to ensure the implementation of actions to prevent NCD risk factors: **2 actions and 5 measures.**

4.3. Cancer registries

4.3.1. Definition of a cancer registry

A cancer registry, also called a population registry, is a means of collecting, storing and interpreting data on cancer patients. It is a medico-administrative structure whose mission is to register all cases of cancer occurring in a defined territory and to ensure the exploitation of the file thus constituted for statistical and epidemiological purposes[(169)].

- **The value of cancer registries in health planning and clinical and epidemiological research :**

The original purpose of morbidity registers was limited to describing the epidemiological situation, studying trends and surveying geographical distribution.

Subsequently, other areas of use of registers will be identified, in particular

- ***contribution to the study of the natural history of diseases, through variations in incidence over time.***
- ***support for needs identification and health planning.***
- ***aids to etiological research:*** The study of the distribution of cancers makes it possible to identify for each type of cancer groups at high risk and others at lower risk.
- ***support for the evaluation of screening and other prevention measures.***

These data are of immense value to the wilaya, the region, the country and for sharing with the world. They provide reliable indications on the cancer profile, indicating incidence, trend and survival rates and allow the improvement of knowledge on cancer in the country[(2)].

4.3.2. History of registers in Algeria

In order to know the epidemiological profile of the cancerous disease in Algeria, from the end of the 1980s, cancer registers were set up in different regions of the country, This made it possible to identify the prevalent neoplastic locations in both men and women and, above all, to initiate a number of actions in the context of the fight against cancer, such as cervical and breast cancer screening campaigns, the erection of new cancer centres, medical training in oncology and the reinforcement of the radiotherapy equipment.

Algeria has gone through several stages:

- Hospital registers: RALAK 1956, Pr. Allouache 1980, Pr. Illoul (13th CMM, 1983).
- Anatomopathological register: Pr. Abdenour Yaker 1975.
- Population registers: Before 2015, there were 17 population registers, including 3 validated by the IARC, that of Setif in the East (first register set up in 1985), Algiers in the Centre (digestive cancer register in 1985, extended to all sites from 1992), and Oran in the West of the country (1994), and registers in the process of consolidation[(170, 171)].

IN 2015, the institutionalisation of the NCCRN:
The national network of registries was created in 2015, within the framework of the 2015 cancer plan 2019[(1)], and its strategic axis number 6 concerning the development of the information and communication system on cancers.
The creation of the network of registers is reinforced by Order No. 22 of 18 February 2014[(10)],

which institutionalised the population registers, with the consolidation of existing registers and the setting up of new registers in all the country's wilayas (11).

This institutionalisation of registers allows us to have a wide registration coverage and therefore reliable incidence data, representative of the whole country, with projections for the coming years.

The aim is to achieve high coverage of cancer registration through the consolidation of existing registries and the establishment of new registries, thereby providing comprehensive and valid national incidence data.

Strategic organisation of the National Cancer Registry Network

- Implementation of Order N°22 of 18 February 20 on the institutionalisation of the registration of Cancer Registries in Algeria[10].
- Conversion into an action of the measure of the strategic axis number 6 concerning the development of the information and communication system on cancer of the National Cancer Plan 2015-2019[1].
- Training of wilaya registry coordinators on Canreg 5 provided by the International Agency for Research on Cancer, and on cancer registration tools
- Monitoring of data collection, data entry, data control, and data analysis.
- Validation of records and data for publication.

Structural organisation of the National Cancer Registry Network

All of the country's wilayas are divided into three regional networks: East and South-East, Central and South-Central and West and South-West, coordinated by the National Cancer Registry Network[170]:

- The East and South East network is coordinated by the Setif Cancer Registry and comprises 20 wilayas: Setif, Annaba, Bejaia, El Taref, Khenchela, Skikda, Souk-Ahras, Biskra, Constantine, Oum El Bouaghi, El Oued, Guelma, Bordj Bou Arreridj (BBA), Tebessa, Jijel, Msila, Batna, Mila, Illizi, Ouargla.
- The Central and South Central network is coordinated by the INSP and comprises 13 wilayas: Algiers, Blida, Medea, Tipaza, Ghardaia, Tizi-Ouzou, Djelfa, Tamanrasset, Ain Defla, Boumerdes, Bouira, Laghouat, Chlef.
- The West and South-West network is coordinated by the Oran Cancer Registry and comprises 15 wilayas: Oran, Mostaganem, Tlemcen, Adrar, Relizane, Tiaret, Mascara, Tissemsilt, Sidi-Bel-Abbes, Tindouf, Naama, Saida, Bechar, Ain Timouchent, Elbayeth.

1. Objectives of the study

- **Main objective:**

The main objective is to study the incidence, geographical distribution and revolution of digestive cancers in the East and South-East region of Algeria.

- **Secondary objectives:**

1. To estimate the incidence of different digestive cancers in the East and South-East region.
2. To determine the evolutionary trend of different digestive cancers in the East and South-East region.
3. Mapping of digestive cancers in the East and South-East region of Algeria.
4. Studying geographical variability.
5. To propose analytical studies on risk factors for digestive cancers specific to the region and avenues for research.
6. To propose recommendations for prevention and screening.

2. Methods

2.1. Type and period of the study :

This is a multicentre cross-sectional epidemiological study of all cases of digestive cancer diagnosed in the eastern and south-eastern regions of Algeria, covering 19 wilayas (Setif, Annaba, Bejaia, El Taref, Khenchela, Skikda, Souk-Ahras, Biskra, Constantine, Oum El Bouaghi, El Oued, Guelma, BBA, Tebessa, Jijel, M'sila, Batna, Mila, Ouargla) from 1er January 2014 to 31 December 2018.

2.2. Target population :

The target population of our study is the one covered by the East and South-East Algerian network (ESEA) except for the wilaya of Illizi (due to the non-functionality of this register).

The East and South-East network covers the population of the 19 wilayas of the East and South-East region of Algeria, the average population estimate in 2017 was 16,826,987 (8,498,113 males and 8,328,873 females), according to the data of the National Statistics Office (ONS)

Description of the East and South-East Algerian region and population: (see Annex I)

2.3. Validation criteria for cancer registries :

- Registries that have received training on cancer registration in regional simulation workshops.

- Registers are in accordance with the ministerial decree relating to the institutionalisation of cancer registers in Algeria.
- Regional and central validation of the quality of the information collected after data entry and control.
- Mastery of cancer registration tools.
- Knowledge of the International Classification of Diseases for Oncology Third Version (ICD O-3).
- The microscopic verification percentage index (the proportion of incident cases with

histological and/or cytological verification of cancer diagnosis) of cases above 90%.

- Respect for the geographical boundaries of each wilaya.
- Duplication and follow-up control of patients.
- consistent quality data for new registers.

2.4. Data collection and management

2.4.1. Registry teams: They are composed of epidemiologists, pathologists and general practitioners at the level of university hospitals and public health establishments.

2.4.2. Collection method: The cancer registries actively collect essential information from cancer patients aged 0-99 years in each wilaya. All information is collected in a standardised form for all types of cancer.

2.4.3. Data sources: the network registers collect data from cancer centres, university hospitals, public hospitals, local public health establishments, public and private anatomopathology laboratories, medical imaging centres and from cancer support associations.

2.4.4. Case definition :

Inclusion criteria: In the present study, all cases of primary cancers are included, namely: cancer of the resophagus, stomach, liver, biliary tract, pancreas, small intestine, colon and rectum; and are domiciled in the different wilayas of the East and South-East Algerian network.

Non-inclusion criteria :

- Subjects not domiciled in the different wilayas of the East and South-East Algerian network.
- Past cases, recurrence and metastasis.
- Cancer in situ.
- Subjects with incomplete information.

2.4.5. Information support, classification and coding :

Data are collected for each new cancer case on a descriptive survey form, using direct coding for some variables at the time of the survey, and central coding for other variables. The coding is done according to the International Classification of Diseases, 3-digit, morphology code according to the International Classification of Diseases for Oncology 3eme revision (ICD O3)[172] . The data includes :

- Personal data (name, surname, sex, date of birth, place of residence);
- The date and basis of diagnosis ;
- Diagnosis (location, morphology) ;
- Follow-up of the patient (living, deceased, date and cause of death);

2.4.6. Registration tools

The registration and verification of registry data is done using Canreg 5 software developed, maintained and provided by the International Agency for Research on Cancer (IARC)/WHO[173] .

2.4.7. Data quality control

A quality control is carried out before the data is recorded on the computer in order to eliminate duplicates and inconsistent cancer cases. A second check is carried out by Canreg5 to verify the internal consistency of the data and their validation. A third check is made once the data entry is completed by the IARC CHECK software provided by IARC[174] .

The validation of the network's overall incidence estimates is based on the estimates obtained between the different registries of the network in a first step, and a second comparison with the estimates made by the IARC on cancer incidences in Algeria (*Globocan* 2018).

2.4.8. Data analysis

The registries in the network use the new version of CANREG 5, developed by the Information Section of the International Agency for Research on Cancer in Lyon.
The in-depth analysis will be done with the *Surveillance Epidemiology And End Results* (SEER*Stat) programme developed by the US National Cancer Institute. The SEER*Stat programme provides a convenient means of analysing the SEER and other international cancer databases. It allows the visualization of individual data and the production of statistics for the study of the impact of cancer on the population, i.e. frequencies, rates, temporal trends. The SEER*Prep program converts the ASCII text files produced by CANREG 5 to the SEER*Stat database.

The incidence data were taken from the incidence tables of the different registers of the network. In this study, the calculation of the overall incidence of the 2014-2018 network is based on the valid registers, i.e. 15 of the 19 existing registers.
The results are presented as the number of registered cases, crude incidence rates, and age-standardised incidence rates (ASR). Age standardisation was performed by the direct method based on the world standard population.
Regional estimates :
- For each location, the crude and standardised incidence rates for the region are estimated from the 15 valid registers, the non-valid registers (for the last 3 years) are excluded, namely those of : Mila, Khenchela, M'sila and Guelma.
Crude incidence rate of the region= Total new cases observed / Total corresponding populations. * expressed per 100 000 inhabitants
Direct standardisation: is used to estimate the standardised incidence rate for the region. The expected new cases are calculated from the standardised incidence rates of each valid register as follows:
Expected cases = standardised incidence rate X registry population.
Region standardised rate = Total expected cases / Total corresponding populations. * expressed per 100,000 inhabitants
Average annual variations :
For both incidence rates and new cases, the average annual change (AAC) between the years 2015 and 2018 (denoted Л1 and A2 respectively) is defined as: A2 = $(1 + AAC)^4$. Л1, i.e. VAM = (Л2/Л1) $/^{14}$ - 1. Expressed as a percentage,
VAM = 100 [(X2/X1)V^4 -1].
Projections of new cases (2018-2025) :
Are calculated from the average annual changes in the number of new cases for all digestive cancers and two locations (colon-rectum and stomach).
The projections are made for the wilayas and the ESEA region.
Other software: EXCEL, SPSS IBM version 21 and Photoline software for the maps The results are presented in the form of a table, a graph and a map (average ASR).

2.5. Confidentiality

The Network Registries adhere to the IACR / CIRC (2004)[175] guidelines for maintaining confidentiality in the process of collecting, storing, using and transmitting identifiable data.

3. Results

3.1. Population data and coverage of the East and South-East Algerian network (ESEA)

3.1.1. The East and South-East region covers (ONS and Atlas of Setif):

- 41.67% of the wilayas of Algeria;
- 38.74% of municipalities ;
- an area of 27.92%;
- a population of 39.02%;

3.1.2. Valid registers in 2017

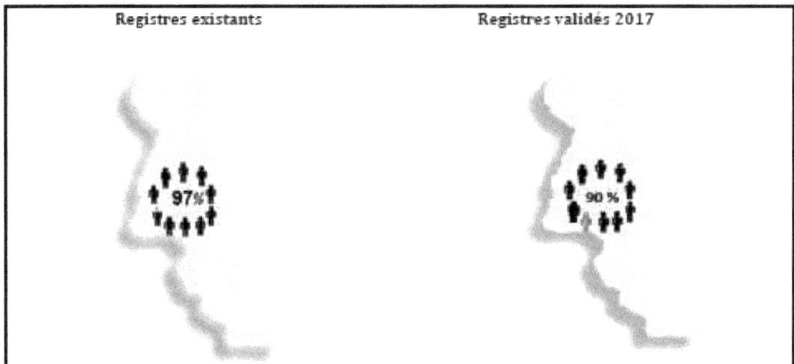

Figure 27. Number of valid registers in the ESEA network, 2017.

Of the 20 existing registers, 19 are valid.

3.1.3. Evolution of cancer case registration in valid ESEA registries 2014 - 2018

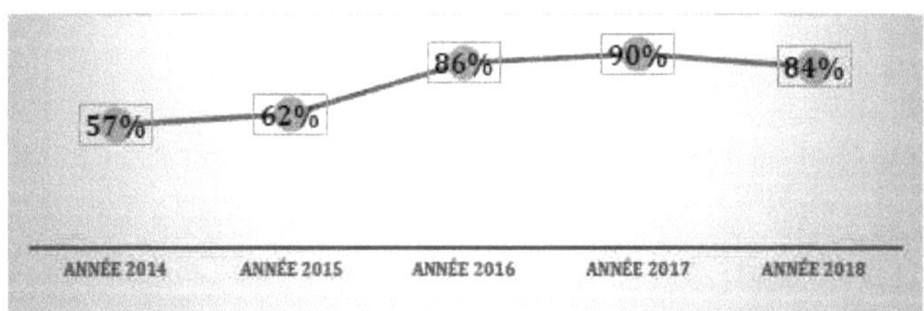

Figure 28. Evolution of cancer registration coverage rates of valid ESEA registries 2014 - 2018.

Population	Masculin	Féminin	Total
Population du Réseau	8 661 679	8 462 566	16 826 987
Population couverte	7 795 511	7 621 709	15 528 870

Table 7: Population covered by cancer registration, East and South-East Network (2017)

Network population	8661679	8 462 566	16 826 987
Population covered	7 795 511	7 621 709	15 528 870

As of 31 December 2017, the cancer registration coverage rate reached 90% of the population of eastern and south-eastern Algeria, i.e. 15,528,870 inhabitants. In 2018, this rate dropped to 84%.

3.2. Overall incidence data (East and South-East network) :

3.2.1. Overall incidence data by gender (East and South-East Network), 2017 :

Table 8: Crude and sex-standardised incidence by location (East and South-East Network, 2017)

	Number of new cases	Gross rate/100,000h	Standardised rate /100 000h
Male	8175	123,6	159,8
Female	10858	162,9	195,4
Total	**19033**	**143,3**	**178,0**

In 2017, the number of new cases for all sites in both sexes was 19033, giving a crude incidence rate of 143.3 per 100,000 population, and standardised to the world population of 178.0 per 100,000.

The incidence of female cancers was higher with 10,858 new cases, a crude rate of 162.9 per 100,000 population and a standardised rate of 195.4 per 100,000 population.

In men the number of new cases was 8175, which corresponds to a crude rate of 123.6 per 100,000 inhabitants and a standardised rate of 159.8 per 100,000 inhabitants.

There is a slight female predominance (sex ratio = 0.75).

3.2.2. Incidence data for the main sites in the East and South East Network for 2017 in women:

Table 9: Crude, standardised incidence and rank of major cancer sites (East and South East Network), year 2017, in women.

location	Number of cases	Gross rate	Standardized rate	% /other cancers
Breast	4126	61,9	73,4	42,4
Colon rectum	1216	14,5	18,3	11,2
Thyroid	713	10,7	12,3	7,7
Uterine cervix	480	4,2	5,5	3,2
Stomach	315	3,8	4,9	2,9
Biliary tract	251	3,0	4,4	2,3

Leukemia	173	2,5	3,0	1,7

The most frequent cancer site in women is breast cancer with a proportion of 42% of cases registered in 2017, which corresponds to a standardised rate of 73.4 per 100 000 inhabitants. CRC ranked second with 11.2% of cases, followed by thyroid and cervical cancer with 7.7% and 3.2% respectively. Next came biliary tract cancer and leukaemia.

3.2.3. Incidence data for the main locations in the East and South-East Network for the year 2017 in men :

Table 10: Crude, standardised incidence and rank of major cancer sites (East and South East Network), year 2017, in men.

location	Number of cases	Gross rate	Standardized rate	%/ to other cancers
Lung and bronchial tubes	1357	17,2	22,0	16,6
Colon rectum	1300	15,2	20,0	15,9
Prostate	1194	13,7	17,9	14,6
Bladder	682	8,5	11,9	8,3
Stomach	521	6,1	8,9	6,4
Leukemia	344	4,2	5,0	4,2
Nasopharynx	321	4,0	5,1	3,9

The most frequent cancer location in men is lung, representing 23% of the cases registered in 2017, which corresponds to a standardised rate of 22 per 100,000 inhabitants, followed by colorectal cancer with a proportion of 15.9% and prostate cancer in third place with 14.6% of cases.

Gastric cancers are in 5eme position among the most frequent male cancers with 6.4%.

3.3. Incidence data for all digestive cancers (East and South East network), 2014 - 2018 :

3.3.1. Proportion of digestive cancers in both sexes (East and South-East network) ,2014 - 2018 :

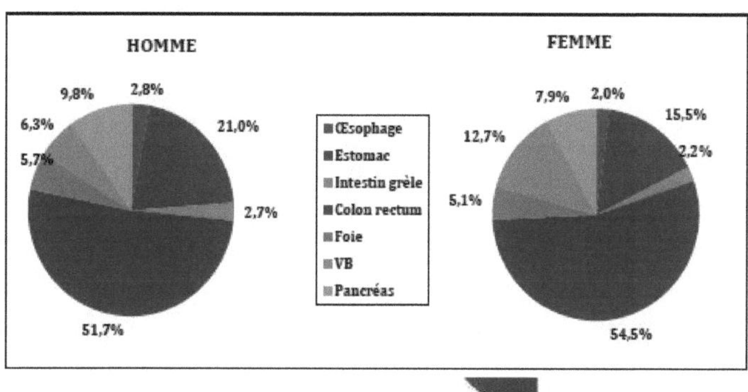

Figure 29. Distribution of digestive cancers in both sexes, East and South-East Network ,2014 - 2018.

CRC ranks first among all digestive cancers in both sexes with 51.7% in men and 54.5% in women, followed by stomach cancer.

In men, it is pancreatic cancer which comes in 3eme position with 9.8% but for women it is extrahepatic biliary cancer with 12.7%.

Cancers of the liver, resophagus and grafted bowel are less common in this region.

3.3.2. Incidence of all digestive cancers in both sexes, East and South East Region 2014-2018:

Table 11. Crude, standardised, mean and rank incidence of all digestive cancers (Reseau Est and Sud- Est), 2014 - 2018 in both sexes.

Year	2014		2015		2016		2017		2018		Average	
Gender	H	F	H	F	H	F	H	F	H	F	H	F
Number of new case	1545	1344	199	1836	2170	1952	2325	2058	2590	2246	10642	9436
Gross rate	19,2	17,1	24,3	22,9	25,9	23,8	27,1	24,5	29,6	26,3	26,8	24,4
Rate Standardised*	26,1	22,1	33,0	29,4	36,6	31,7	39,0	33,3	40,2	34,1	37,2	32,2
% / others cancers	26,8	18,1	28,2	17,0	27,7	19,3	30,4	19,6	31,0	19,9	28,8	18,8

There has been a marked increase in the number of new cases of digestive cancers, with 20078 cases recorded during 2014 - 2018 with a slight male predominance (sex ratio = 1.13).

The mean crude incidence was 26.8 in men and 24.4 in women, which corresponds to standardised rates of 37.2 and 32.2 respectively.

Digestive cancers represent on average 28.8% of male cancers and 18.8% of female cancers.

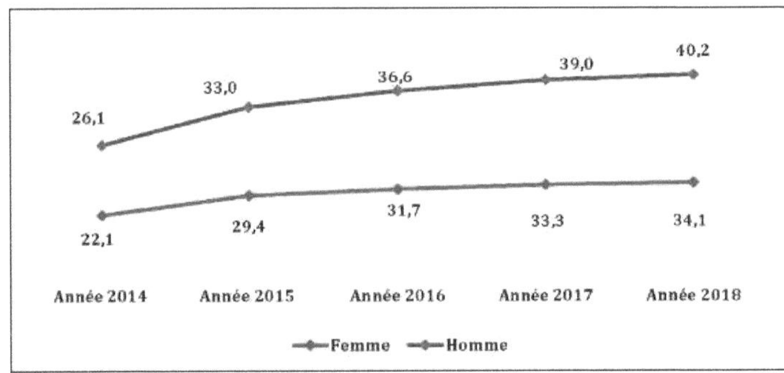

Figure 30. Trend in standardised incidence of digestive cancers in both sexes, East and South-East region, 2014 - 2018.

There was a rapid increase in ASR incidence between 2014 and 2015 and then a slower increase of 2 per 100,000 population per year for both sexes.

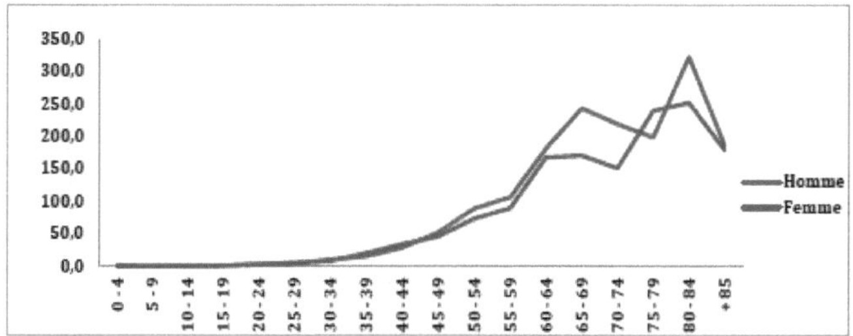

Figure 31. Distribution of standardised digestive cancer rates by age group and sex, ESEA region 2017.

3.3.3. Incidence of digestive cancers according to age :

94% of digestive cancers occur after the age of 40. The median age is 62 years for both sexes.

The specific incidence rates increase progressively in both sexes, reaching a peak between 65 and 70 years of age (243.8 per 100,000 men and 171.3 per 100,000 women) and a second peak after 80 years of age.

3.3.4. Geographical variations in the incidence of digestive cancers

3.3.4.1. Standardised incidences of some ESEA registers, 2017

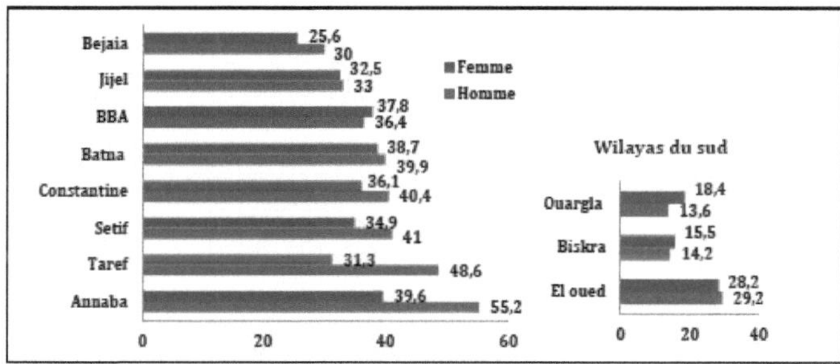

Figure 32. Comparison of standardised incidences of digestive cancers in some registries of the East and South-East network, 2017.

In men, the highest incidence of digestive cancers in 2017 was recorded in Annaba (55.2), El Taref (48.6), Setif (41.0) and Constantine (40.4). Among women, the wilayas most concerned are Annaba (39.6), Batna (38.7) and BBA (37.8).

The registers in the south-east have a lower incidence rate than those in the north, the highest being that of El Oued (29.2 per 100 000 men and 28.2 per 100 000 women).

3.3.4.2. Geographical variation in the mean incidence of digestive cancers in both sexes.

Table 12. Distribution of number of cases, mean crude and standardised incidence, of all digestive cancers according to the different East and South-East Network registries in men, 2014 - 2018.

Register	Total number of cases	Average gross rate*.	Standardised rate medium*.
Annaba	794	51,7	57,2
Jijel	440	25,1	42,1
El Taref	214	28,7	40,6
Batna	723	21,9	36,8
Setif	1051	24,6	36,4
Bejaia	662	25,7	35,8
Souk-Ahras	218	27,0	35,7
Constantine	782	28,8	35,5
BBA	397	21,2	32,4
El Oued	237	18,9	31,4
Skikda	391	18,0	23,6
Biskra	227	11,4	22,3
Oum El Bouaghi	264	17,2	21,5
Ouargla	167	10,4	18,4
Tebessa	138	11,5	17,1
East and South-East Region	**10642**	**26,8**	**37,2**

In men, the wilaya of Setif recorded the highest number of digestive cancer cases (1051 cases) during the period 2014 - 2018, followed by Annaba, Constantine, Batna and Bejaia.
The wilayas of : Annaba, Jijel and El Taref had a higher average crude and standardised incidence than the region. The wilaya of Annaba had a remarkably high incidence of 57.2 per 100 000 inhabitants.
The wilayas of Setif, Constantine, Bejaia and Souk-Ahras had an incidence close to that of the region. It varies between 36.8 and 35.5.

BBA and EL oued recorded respectively lower rates than the region 32.4 and 31.4 per 100 000 inhabitants
The other wilayas recorded low, or even very low, incidence rates, such as the wilayas of Ouargla and Tebessa.

Table 13. Distribution of number of cases, mean crude and standardised incidence, of all digestive cancers according to the different East and South-East registries in women, 2014 - 2018.

Register	Total number of cases	Average gross rate*.	Standardised rate medium*.
Annaba	622	40,1	44,3
Jijel	448	25,6	40,5

Batna	717	22,3	37,0
Setif	996	24,8	33,2
BBA	420	23,1	33,2
Bejaia	557	23,3	28,3
El Taref	154	20,7	27,9
Constantine	672	24,8	27,8
El Oued	193	16,0	27,5
Souk-Ahras	162	20,0	25,5
Skikda	340	15,9	21,1
Ouargla	155	9,9	19,1
Biskra	206	10,4	18,2
Oum El Bouaghi	234	15,6	18,0
Tebessa	135	11,4	17,8
East and South East Region	**9436**	**24,4**	**32,2**

In women, the number of cases was the same as in men. However, in terms of incidence, the wilayas of Annaba, Jijel, Batna, Setif and BBA recorded the highest rates.

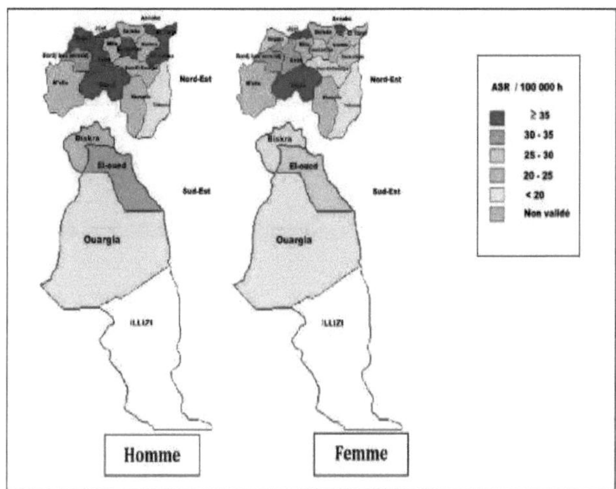

Figure 33. Mapping of all digestive cancers, ESEA region 2014 - 2018.

3.4. Incidence data by location of digestive cancers (East and South-East network), 2014 - 2018 :

3.4.1. Colorectal cancer (CRC)

3.4.1.1. Incidence of colorectal cancer (ICD-10: C18-C21) (East and South-East network), 2014-2018

Table 14: Crude, standardised, mean and rank incidence of CRC in both sexes (East and South East Network), 2014 - 2018.

Year	2014		2015		2016		2017		2018		Average	
Gender	H	F	H	F	H	F	H	F	H	F	H	F
Number of new case	775	727	1048	1018	1124	1085	1300	1216	1469	1330	5673	5377

Gross rate	9,6	9,3	12,8	12,7	13,4	13,2	15,2	14,5	16,8	15,6	14,6	14,0
Rate Standardise*	13,5	12,3	17,7	16,8	18,6	17,7	20,5	19,0	21,9	21,1	19,3	18,2
% / other cancers	13,4	8,4	14,8	9,4	14,3	9,9	15,9	11,2	17,6	11,8	15,9	11,2

CRC is the leading digestive cancer in both men and women. The number of new cases of CRC registered from 01 January 2014 to 31 December 2018 is 11050 cases, affecting men 1.1 times more than women.

In men, these cancers have increased significantly from a crude incidence rate of 9.6 and a standardised incidence rate of 13.5 per 100,000 population in 2014, to a crude incidence rate of 16.8 and a standardised incidence rate of 21.9 per 100,000 population in 2018.
In both women and men there has been a clear increase in crude or standardised incidence rates.

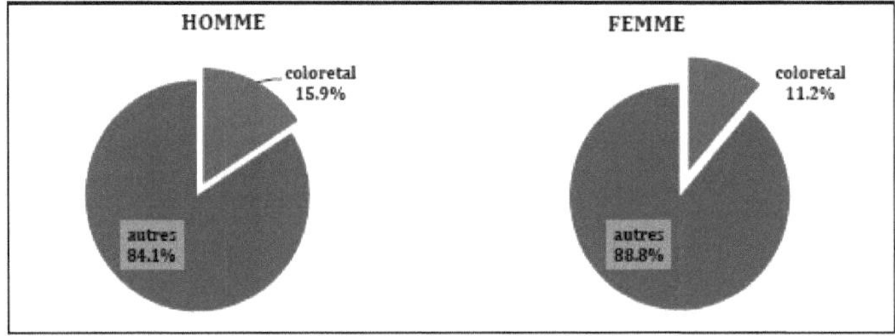

Figure 34: The share of colorectal cancers among all cancers in both sexes, Region ESEA 2014 - 2018.

CRC accounted for 15.9% of male cancer cases and 11.2% of female cancers between 2014 and 2018.

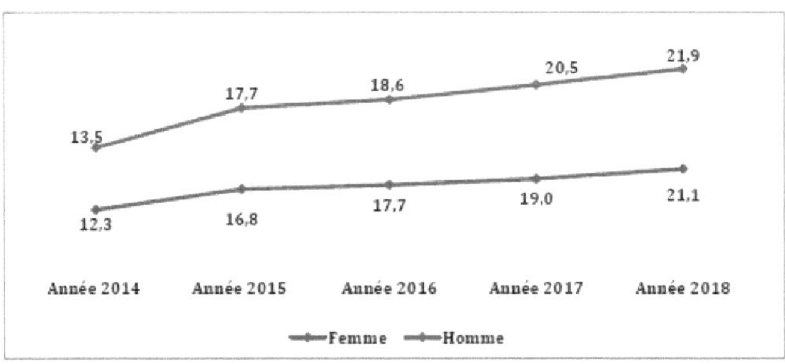

Figure 35. The share of colorectal cancers among all cancers in both sexes, Region ESEA 2014 - 2018.

There was a rapid increase in incidence ASR between 2014 and 2015 and then a less rapid increase in both sexes (VAM = 6% between 2015 and 2018).

3.4.1.2. Variations in colorectal cancer incidence by age (East and South-East Network), 2017

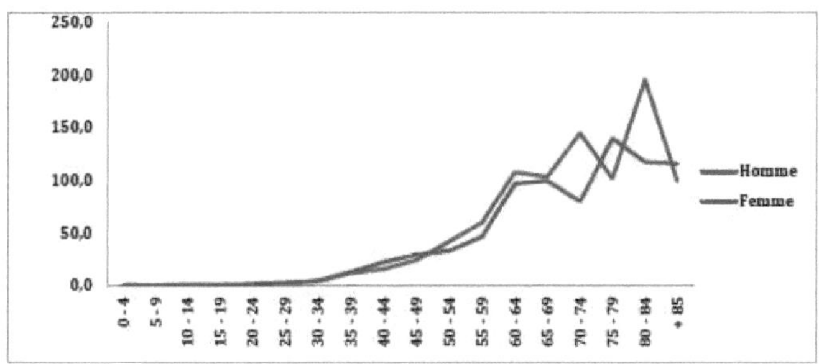

Figure 36. Distribution of standardised CRC rates by age and sex, ESEA region 2017.

The specific incidence of CRC increases with age in both sexes. The median age at diagnosis in 2017 was 63 years for men and 62 years for women. meThe cross-sectional curve of incidence rates according to age shows a marked progression of rates from the age of 45 (91.3% of cases) in both sexes to reach a maximum value of 144.5 in men between 70 and 74 years of age and 99.4 in women between 65 and 69 years of age, followed by a peak of 195.5 in men between 80 and 84 years of age and 117.2 in women between 75 and 79 years.

3.4.1.3. Geographical variations in the incidence of RCCs

3.4.1.3.1 Standardized CRC incidences of selected ESEA registries, 2017

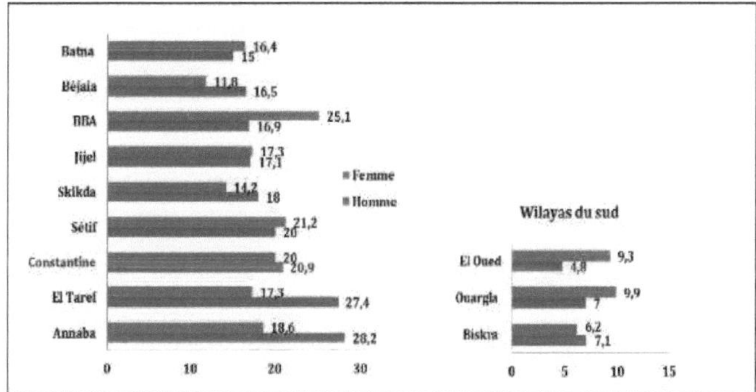

Figure 37. Comparison of standardised CRC cancer incidences of some registries in the East and South-East network, 2017.

In 2017, in men, the highest incidence of CRC was recorded in Annaba (28.2), El Taref (27.4), Constantine (20.9) and Skikda (18.0). Among women, the most affected wilayas were BBA (25.1), Setif (21.2), Constantine (20.0) and Batna (16.4).

The registers in the South-East have recorded lower incidence rates than those in the North. The highest rates are observed in Ouargla and there is a predominance of female CRCs in the south.

3.4.1.3.2. Geographical variations in the average incidence of colorectal cancers in both sexes.

Table 15. Distribution of the number of cases, mean crude and standardised incidence, of CRC according to the different registries of the Reseau Est and Sud-Est in men, 2014 - 2018.

Register	Total number of cases	Average gross rate*.	Average standardised* rate
Annaba	402	26,1	28,4
Jijel	222	12,7	21,1
El Taref	106	14,2	19,7
Setif	577	13,7	19,6
Bejaia	355	13,9	19,3
Constantine	420	15,2	18,8
BBA	208	11,0	16,5
Batna	303	9,3	15,3
Souk-Ahras	89	11,0	14,1
Skikda	227	10,4	13,4
El Oued	111	8,9	12,9
Oum El Bouaghi	145	9,4	11,6
Biskra	108	5,6	11,4
Ouargla	95	6,0	10,2
Tebessa	59	4,9	7,2
East and South East Region	**5673**	**14,6**	**19,3**

In humans, the wilaya of Setif recorded the highest number of CRC cases (577 cases) during the period 2014 - 2018, followed by Constantine, Annaba, Bejaia and Batna.

The wilayas of Annaba, Jijel, El Taref, Setif and Bejaia had a higher standardised average incidence than those in the region. The wilaya of Annaba has a remarkably high incidence of 28.2 per 100,000 inhabitants.

The average rates in Constantine (18.8) and Bejaia (19.3) were close to those of the region. BBA and Batna recorded respectively lower rates than the region and 16.5 and 15.3 per 100 000 inhabitants.

The other wilayas had low, or even very low, incidence rates, such as the wilayas of Tebessa and Ouargla.

Table 16. Distribution of the number of cases, mean crude and standardised incidence, of CRC according to the different registries of the East and South-East Network in women, 2014 - 2018.

Register	Total number of case	Average gross rate*.	Standardized rate medium
Annaba	334	21,3	23,8
Jijel	235	13,2	21,0
BBA	253	14,0	20,1
Setif	580	14,7	19,1
Constantine	395	14,7	16,3
Batna	329	10.2	15,8
El Taref	79	10,6	14,3
Bejaia	264	10,7	12,9
Skikda	192	9,0	11,6
El Oued	78	6,5	10,9
Ouargla	84	5,5	10,4
Souk-Ahras	66	8,2	10,1
Tebessa	78	6,6	10,1
Oum El Bouaghi	114	7,6	8,6
Biskra	77	4,0	6,7
East and South-East Region	**5377**	**14,0**	**18,2**

In women, the number of cases is the same. However, in terms of incidence, the wilayas of Annaba, Jijel, Setif and BBA recorded the highest rates.

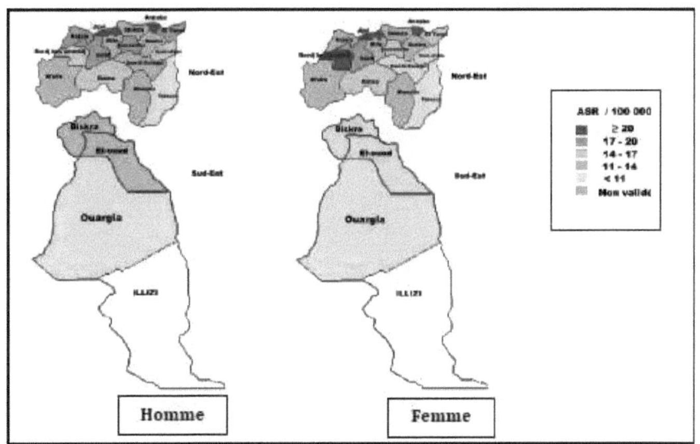

Figure 38. Mapping of ACCs, ESEA region 2014 - 2018.

3.4.2. Stomach cancer

3.4.2.1. Incidence of gastric cancer (ICD-10: C16) (East and South East network), 2014-2018

Table 17: Crude, standardised, mean and rank incidence of stomach cancer in both sexes (East and South East Network), 2014 - 2018.

Year	2014		2015		2016		2017		2018		Average	
Gender	H	F	H	F	H	F	H	F	H	F	H	F
Number of new case	318	232	455	291	470	338	521	315	555	355	2319	1531
Gross rate	4,0	2,9	5,5	3,6	5,6	4,1	6,1	3,8	6,3	4,1	5,9	3,9
Standardized rate	5,4	3,9	7,6	4,7	8,1	5,6	9,0	5,1	8,8	5,3	8,2	5,1
% / other Cancers	5,5	3,1	6,4	2,7	6,1	3,3	6,4	2,9	6,6	3,1	6,0	3,1

meStomach cancer is the 2nd most common digestive cancer in men and women.
The number of new cases of stomach cancer recorded in 2018 was 910 cases, and the cumulative number of cases since 2014 was 3850 cases, of which 60.1% were in men. It affects men 1.6 times more than women.

In men, the incidence rate is stable with periods of slight non-significant increase, in 2014 the crude rate was 4.0 and the standardised incidence rate was 5.4 per 100,000 population, in 2018 the crude incidence rate was 6.3 and the standardised incidence rate is 8.8 per 100,000 population
In women the evolution is identical.

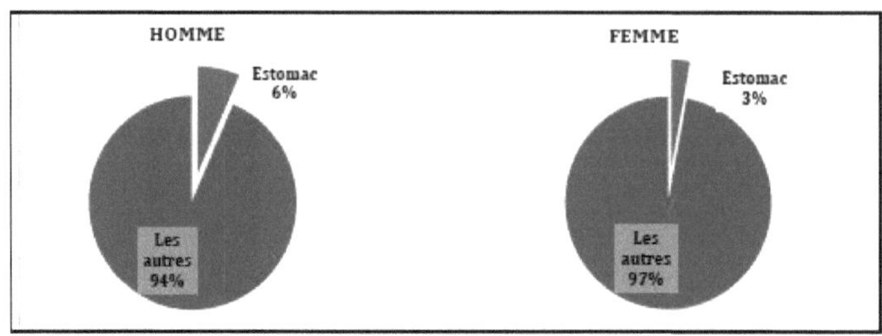

Figure 39. The share of gastric cancers among all cancers in both sexes, ESEA Network 2014 - 2018.

Gastric cancers represent 6% of male cancer cases and 11.2% of female cancers between 2014 and 2018.

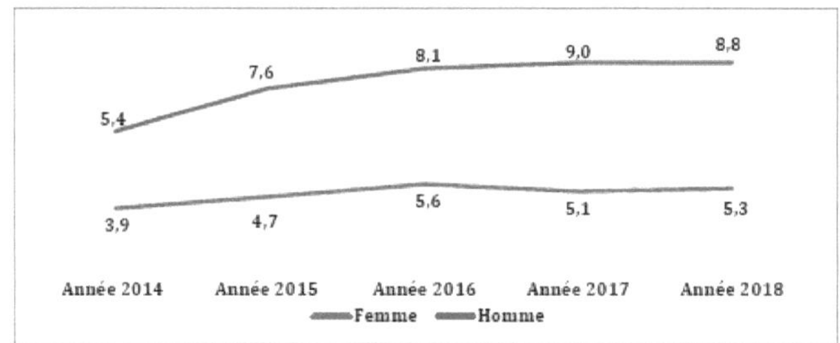

Figure 40: Trend in standardised incidence of gastric cancer in both sexes, East and South-East region, 2014 - 2018.

Between 2014 and 2016, the standardised rate increased significantly from 5.4 in men and 3.9 per 100,000 inhabitants in women to 8.1 in men and 5.6 in women. It then stabilises and remains between 7.5 and 9 in men and 4.5 and 5.3 in women respectively. Variations in the incidence of gastric cancer according to age (East and South-East network), 2017

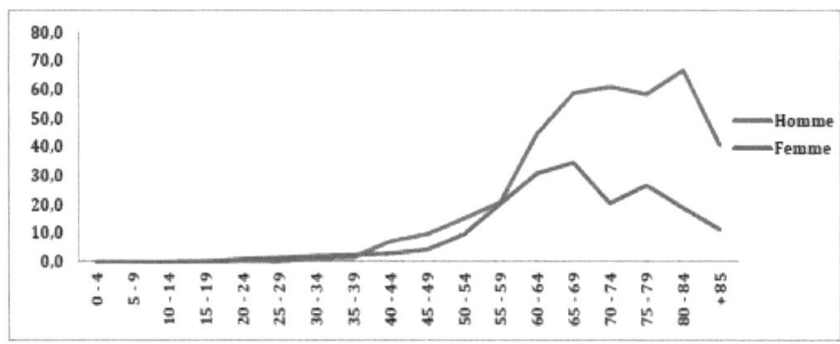

Figure 41. Distribution of standardised gastric cancer rates by age and sex, ESEA region 2017.

The specific incidence of gastric cancer increases with age in both sexes. In 2017, the median age at diagnosis was 67 years for men and 62 years for women. meThe cross-sectional curve of incidence rates according to age shows a marked progression of rates from the age of 40 (95% of cases) in both sexes, reaching a maximum value of 58.9 in men and 34.7 in women between 65 and 69 years of age, followed by a peak of 66.8 in men between 80 and 84 years of age and 26.8 in women between 75 and 79 years of age.

3.4.2.2. Geographical variations in the incidence of gastric cancer

3.4.2.2.1. Standardised incidence of gastric cancer in selected ESEA registries, 2017

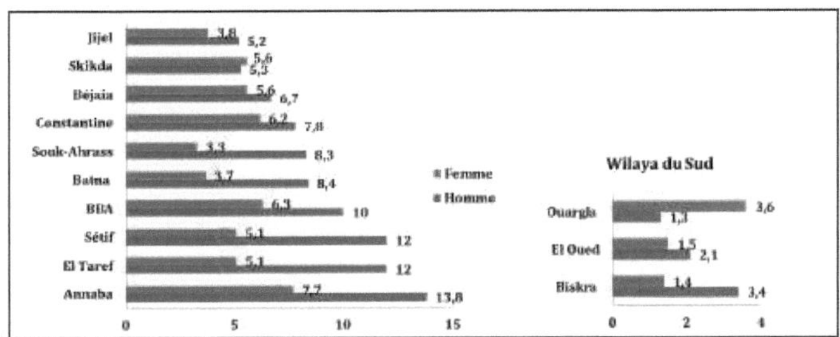

Figure 42. Comparison of standardised incidences of gastric cancer in some registries of the East and South-East network, 2017.

In men, in 2017, the highest incidence of stomach cancer was recorded in Annaba (13.8), El Taref (12.0), Setif (12.0) BBA (10.0) and Batna (8.4). Among women, the wilayas most affected were Annaba (7.7), BBA (6.3) and Constantine (6.2).

The registers in the south-east recorded lower incidence rates than those in the north. The highest incidence in men is observed in Biskra and in Ouargla in women.

The majority of wilayas are male-dominated, except for Skikda and Biskra.

3.4.2.2.2. Geographical variations in the mean incidence of gastric cancer in both sexes.

Table 18. Distribution of the number of cases, mean crude and standardised incidence, of gastric cancers according to the different registries of the East and South-East Network in men, 2014 - 2018.

Register	Total number of cases	Average gross rate*.	Average standardised* rate
Annaba	201	13	14,9
El Taref	52	7,0	9,8
BBA	118	6,2	9,7
Constantine	188	6,9	8,3
Setif	223	5,4	8,2
Bejaia	136	5,4	7,4
Souk-Ahras	44	5,4	7,4
Batna	136	4,3	7,3
Jijel	74	4,0	7,1
Skikda	74	3,4	4,6
Tebessa	37	3,1	4,6
Oum El Bouaghi	45	3,0	3,9
Biskra	37	1,9	3,7
El Oued	25	2,0	3,5
Ouargla	29	1,6	2,8

East and South East Region	2319	5,9	8,2

In men, the wilaya of Setif recorded the highest number of stomach cancer cases (223 cases) during the period 2014 - 2018 followed by Annaba, Constantine, Bejaia and Batna.
The wilayas of Annaba, El Taref, BBA and Constantine had a higher average crude and standardised incidence than the region. The wilaya of Annaba had a remarkably high incidence of 14.9 per 100,000 inhabitants.

The average standardised rates in Setif, Bejaia, Souk-Ahras, Batna and Jijel are similar to those in the region.
BBA and Batna recorded respectively lower rates than the region (16.5 and 15.3 per 100 000 inhabitants).
The other wilayas recorded low incidence rates of between 4.6 and 2.8.

Table 19. Distribution of the number of cases, mean crude and standardised incidence, of gastric cancer according to the different registries of the East and South-East Network in women, 2014 - 2018.

Register	Total number of case	Average gross rate	Standardised rate medium
Annaba	116	7,5	8,1
BBA	70	4,1	5,9
El Taref	29	3,9	5,5
Setif	159	3,8	5,1
Bejaia	100	4,3	5,0
Constantine	112	4,1	4,7
Batna	100	3,1	4,7
Jijel	56	3,1	4,7
Skikda	61	2,9	3,8
Ouargla	26	1,8	3,4
Souk-Ahras	22	2,7	3,4
Biskra	32	1,7	3,2
Oum El Bouaghi	40	2,7	2,8
Tebessa	15	1,3	1,8
El Oued	9	0,7	1,2
East and South-East Region	**1531**	**3,9**	**5,1**

In women, the number of cases was the same as in men. However, in terms of incidence, the wilayas of Annaba, BBA, El Taref, Setif and Bejaia recorded the highest rates.

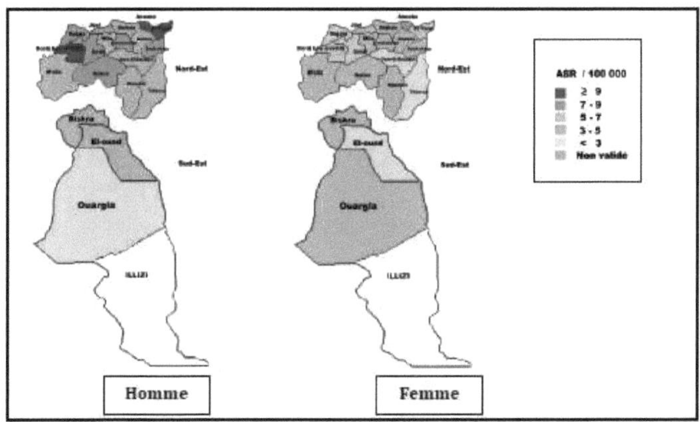

Figure 43. Mapping of gastric cancers, ESEA region 2014 - 2018.

3.4.3. Biliary tract cancers

3.4.3.1 Incidence of VB and extrahepatic biliary tract (EABT) cancers (ICD-10: C23 - 24) (East and South-East network), 2014-2018

Table 20: Crude, standardised, mean and rank incidence of BV and HVLB cancer in both sexes (East and South East Network), 2014 - 2018.

Year	2014		2015		2016		2017		2018		Average	
Gender	H	F	H	F	H	F	H		FH		FH	F
Number of new case	84	190	155	245	138	272	152		251166		298696	1256
Gross rate	1.0	2.4	1,9	3,0	1,6	3,3	1,8		3,01,9	3,5	1,8	3,2
Rate Standardise*	1,6	3,6	2,8	4,3	3,1	5,0	2,5		4,62,8	4,9	3,1	4,6
% / other cancers	1,5	2,6	2,2	2,2	1,6	3,3	1,9	2,3	2,0	2,6	1,9	2,3

Cancer of the VB and VBEH ranks 3®me among digestive cancers in women and 4®me in men.
The number of new cases of BV cancer recorded in 2018 was 464, and the cumulative number of cases since 2014 was 1952, 64% of which were women. There is a predominance of women with a sex ratio of 0.55.

In women, the incidence is increasing, in 2014 the crude rate was 2.4 with a standardised rate of 3.5 per 100,000 population, in 2018 the crude and standardised incidence rate were 3.6 and 4.9 per 100,000 population. In men, a smaller increase is observed.

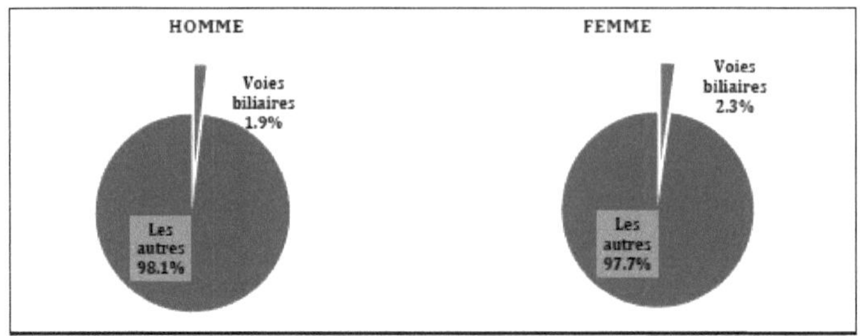

Figure 44. The share of biliary tract cancers among all cancers in both sexes, ESEA Network 2014 - 2018.

meVB cancer is the 6th most common cancer in women, accounting for 2.3% of all cancers in women and only 1.9% of all cancers in men.

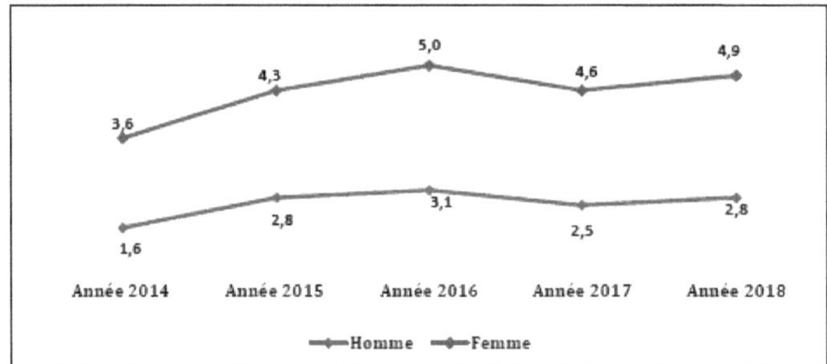

Figure 46. Trend in standardised incidence of biliary tract cancer in both sexes, East and South-East region, 2014 - 2018.

There was a rapid increase in incidence ASRs between 2014 and 2016 until they reached a maximum of 5.0 in women and 3.1 in men, then they decreased in 2017 and in 2018 they were 4.9 in men and 2.8 in women.

3.4.3.2. Variations in the incidence of BV and HVLB cancers according to Age (East and South East Network), 2017

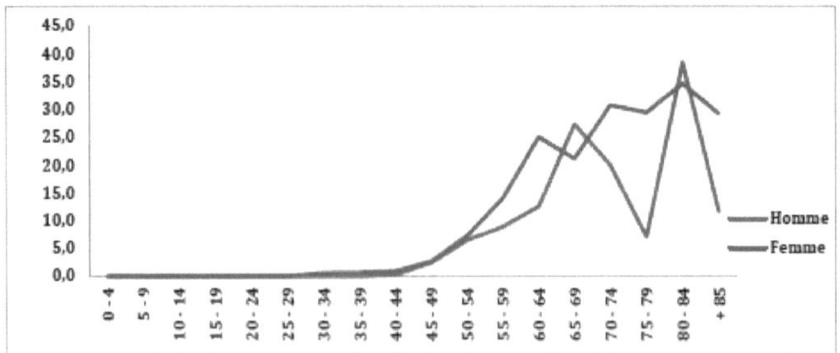

Figure 47. Distribution of standardised biliary tract cancer rates by age and sex, ESEA region

2017

The specific incidence of HNV cancers increases with age in both sexes. The median age at diagnosis in 2017 was 67 years for men and 62 years for women. meThe cross-sectional curve of incidence rates according to age shows a marked progression of rates from the age of 45 (95% of cases) in both sexes to reach a maximum value of 30.8 in women between 70 and 74 years of age and 27.4 in men between 65 and 69 years of age, followed by a peak of 34.7 in women and 38.5 in men between 80 and 84 years of age, with a reversal of the sex ratio in this age group.

3.4.3.3. Geographical variations in the incidence of BV and HVLB cancers

3.4.3.3.1. Standardized incidences of biliary tract cancers from selected ESEA registries, 2017

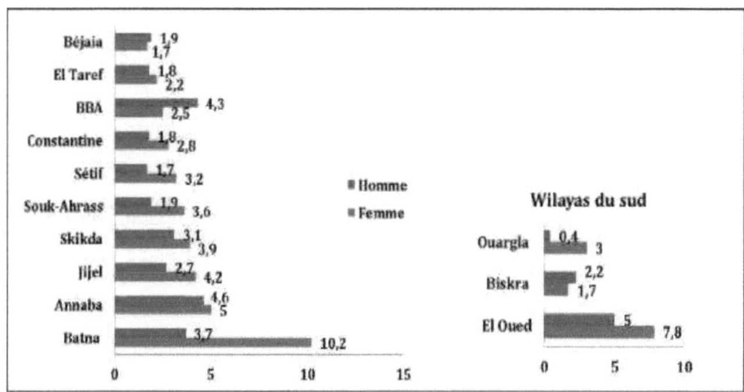

Figure 47. Comparison of standardised incidences of biliary tract cancers from some registries in the East and South-East network, 2017.

In women, in 2017, the incidence of HBEV cancer was remarkably high in Batna (10.2), followed by El Oued (7.8). The other wilayas recorded incidences between 5.0 and 1.7. While in men, the wilayas most concerned are Annaba (4.6), BBA (4.3) and El Oued (5.0).
The registers in the South-East recorded lower incidence rates than those in the North except for El Oued.
The predominance of women is observed in the majority of wilayas except for BBA, Bejaia and Biskra.

3.4.3.3.2. Geographical variations in the mean incidence of biliary tract cancers in both sexes.

Table 21. Distribution of the number of cases, mean crude and standardised incidence, of biliary tract cancers according to the different registries of the East and South-East Network in women, 2014 - 2018.

Register	Total number of cases	Average gross rate*.	Average standardised* rate
El Oued	54	4,5	8,1
Jijel	82	4,9	7,8
Batna	133	4,1	7,3
Annaba	76	5,0	5,6
Souk-Ahras	24	3,0	4,2
Bejaia	74	3,2	4,0
Setif	118	2,8	4,0

Biskra	38	1,9	3,6
Ouargla	20	1,4	3,3
Oum El Bouaghi	33	2,2	2,9
BBA	43	2,0	2,8
Skikda	41	1,9	2,7
El Taref	12	1,6	2,3
Constantine	50	1,6	1,9
Tebessa	9	0,8	1,3
East and South-East Region	**865**	**3,2**	**4,6**

In women, the wilaya of Batna recorded a significant number of cases of VB cancer (133 cases) during the period 2014 - 2018 followed by Annaba, Constantine, Bejaia and Batna.

The wilayas of El Oued, Jijel and Batna had a higher average crude and standardised incidence than the region. The wilaya of El Oued had a remarkably high incidence of 8.1 per 100 000 inhabitants.

The average standardised rates in Annaba, Bejaia, Souk-Ahras and Setif were close to those of the region.

The other wilayas recorded medium-low incidence rates of between 3.6 and 2.3.

The wilaya of Constantine has recorded a low rate of VBEH cancers.

Table 22. Distribution of the number of cases, mean crude and standardised incidence, of biliary tract cancers according to the different registries of the East and South-East Network in men, 2014 - 2018.

Register	Total number of case	Average gross rate*.	Average standardised* rate
Jijel	44	2,6	4,5
Annaba	56	3,8	4,2
El Oued	25	2,0	3,7
El Taref	17	2,3	3,6
Batna	64	2,0	3,5
BBA	25	1,5	2,5
Bejaia	36	1,4	2,2
Souk-Ahras	13	1,6	2,2
Setif	54	1,2	2,0
Constantine	34	1,4	1,9
Biskra	20	0,9	1,8
Skikda	25	1,2	1,7
Oum El Bouaghi	14	0,9	1,3
Ouargla	6	0,4	0,8
Tebessa	6	0,5	0,8
East and South East Region	**467**	**1,8**	**3,1**

In men, the number of cases is the same as for women. The wilayas of Annaba, BBA, El Taref, Setif and Bejaia recorded high rates.

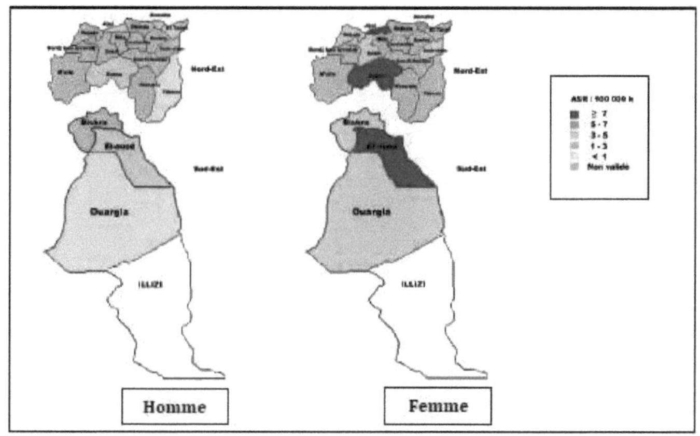

Figure 48. Mapping of biliary tract cancers, ESEA region 2014 - 2018.

3.4.4 Pancreatic cancers

3.4.4.1. Incidence of pancreatic cancers (ICD-10: C25) (Reseau Est and Sud - Est), 2014-2018.

Table 23: Crude, standardised, mean and rank incidence of pancreatic cancer in both sexes (East and South East Network), 2014 - 2018.

Year	2014		2015		2016		2017		2018		Average	
Gender	H	F	H	F	H	F	H	F	H	F	H	F
Number of new case	168	96	144	122	232	175	267	193	272	196	1084	782
Gross rate	2,1	1,2	1,8	1,5	2,8	2,1	3,1	2,3	3,1	2,3	2,7	2,1
Rate Standardise*	3,1	1,6	2,6	2,0	4,2	2,5	5,0	3,2	4,7	3,5	4,0	2,8
% / other cancers	2,9	1,3	2,0	1,1	2,9	1,5	3,3	1,8	3,3	1,7	3,3	1,8

There were an estimated 468 new cases of pancreatic cancer in the region in 2018, 58% of which were in men. emePancreatic cancer accounts for 9.8% of all digestive cancers and is the third most common cancer in men and the fourth most common in women.

The average crude and standardised incidence rates (between 2015 and 2018) were 2.7 and 4.0 cases per 100,000 population for men and 2.1 and 2.8 cases per 100,000 for women (male/female ratio equal to 1.4).

Crude rates increase for both sexes from 2.1 in 2014 to 3.1 in 2018 for men and from 1.2 in 2014 to 2.3 in 2018 for women.

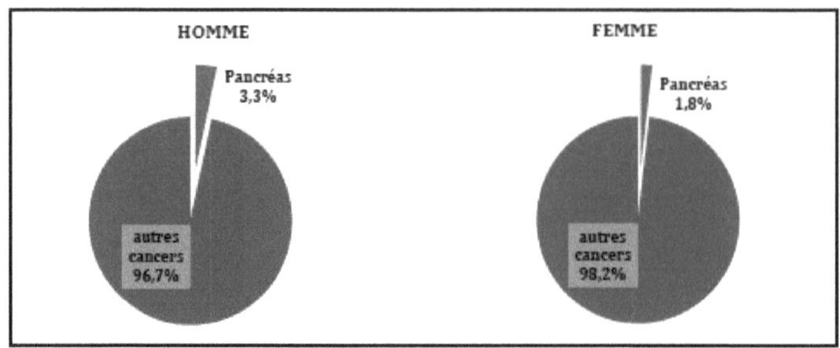

Figure 49. The share of pancreatic cancers among all cancers in both sexes, ESEA region 2014 - 2018.

mePancreatic cancer is the 8th most common cancer in men, accounting for 3.3% of all male cancers and only 1.8% of female cancers.

In men, there is a decrease in incidence ASRs between 2014 and 2015 to a minimum of 2.6 and then they double in 2018. In women, however, they are gradually increasing.

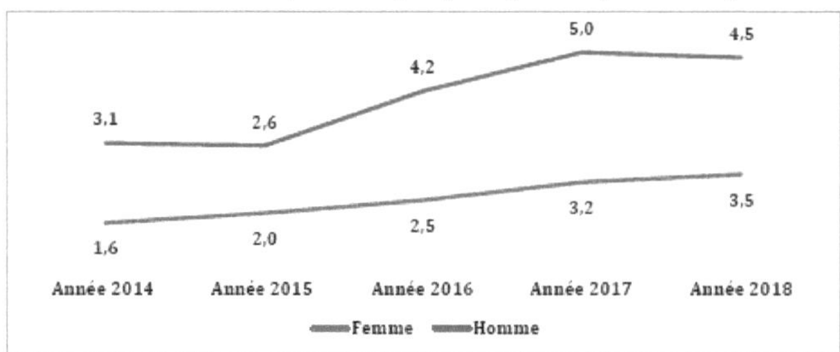

Figure 50. trend in standardised incidence of pancreatic cancer in both sexes, east and south-east region, 2014 - 2018.

3.4.4.2. Variations in the incidence of pancreatic cancer by age (East and South-East network), 2017

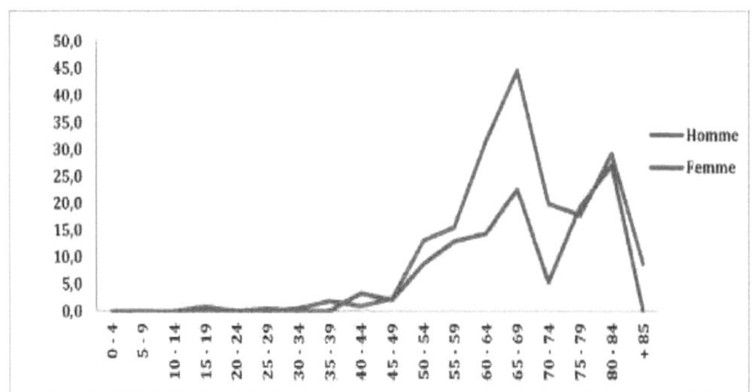

Figure 51. Distribution of standardised pancreatic cancer rates by age and sex, ESEA region 2017.

The median age at diagnosis in 2017 was 63 for men and 62 for women. The cross-sectional curve of incidence rates according to age shows a marked progression of incidence rates from the age of 50 onwards in both sexes, reaching a maximum value of 44.6 in men and 22.6 in women per 100,000 between the ages of 65 and 69, followed by a 2®me peak between the ages of 80 and 84.

3.4.4.3. Geographical variations in the incidence of pancreatic cancer

3.4.4.3.1 Standardized impacts of some ESEA registers, 2017

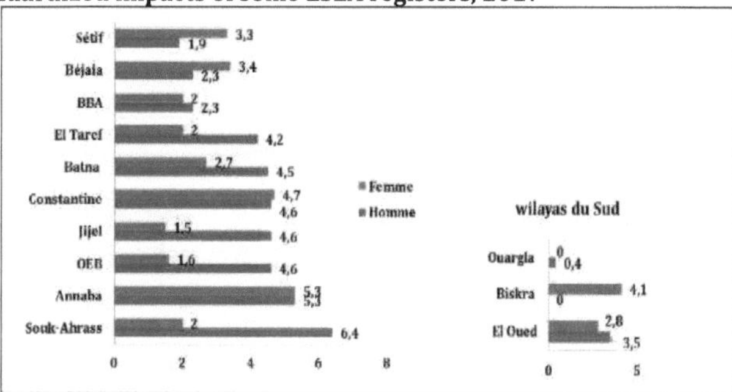

Figure 52. Comparison of standardised incidences of pancreatic cancers in some registries of the East and South-East network, 2017.

In men, in 2017, the highest incidence of pancreatic cancer was recorded in Souk-Ahras (6.4), Annaba (5.3), Jijel and OEB (4.6). In women, the wilayas most concerned are Annaba (5.3. Sex ratio= 1), Constantine (4.7), Biskra (4.1) and Bejaia (3.4).

In 2017, the wilaya of Ouargla recorded only one case of pancreatic cancer.

3.4.4.3.2. Geographical variations in the average incidence of pancreatic cancer in both sexes.

Tableau 24. Distribution of number of cases, mean crude and standardised incidence, of pancreatic cancers according to the different registries of the East and South-East Network in men, 2014 - 2018.

Register	Total number of cases	Average gross rate*.	Average standardised* rate
Souk-Ahras	38	4,7	6,7
Batna	118	3,4	5,9
Jijel	50	3,0	4,9
Annaba	60	4,0	4,5
El Taref	22	3,0	4,2
Constantine	78	3,0	3,7
El Oued	23	1,8	3,5
Bejaia	62	2,3	3,3
Oum El Bouaghi	37	2,4	3,1
Setif	76	1,7	2,7
Tebessa	16	1,3	2,2
BBA	23	1,2	2,0
Skikda	30	1,4	1,8
Biskra	22	1,0	1,7
Ouargla	10	0,6	1,3
East and South-East Region	**1084**	**2,7**	**4,0**

In men, it is the wilaya of Batna that recorded a significant number of pancreatic cancer cases

(118 cases) during the period 2014 - 2018 followed by Constantine and Setif.

The wilayas of Souk-Ahras, Batna, Jijel, Annaba and El Taref had a higher average crude and standardised incidence than the region. The standardised mean rates of Constantine, El Oued and Bejaia were close to those of the region.

The other wilayas have medium-low incidence rates of between 3.1 and 2.0.

The wilayas of the South East have a low incidence of pancreatic cancer.

Tableau 25. Distribution of number of cases, mean crude and standardised incidence, of pancreatic cancers according to the different registries of the East and South-East Network in women, 2014 - 2018.

Register	Total number of cases	Average gross rate*.	Average standardised* rate
Souk-Ahras	22	2,7	3,6
Batna	65	2,1	3,5
Bejaia	63	2,7	3,4
El Oued	22	1,8	3,3
Constantine	69	2,7	3,1
Annaba	45	2,8	3,0
Jijel	32	1,8	2,6
Setif	65	1,7	2,6
Biskra	25	1,3	2,2
BBA	22	1,3	1,8
El Taref	11	1,5	1,7
Oum el Bouaghi	19	1,3	1,6
Tebessa	11	0,9	1,6
Skikda	19	0,9	1,2
Ouargla	10	0,4	0,9
East and South East Region	**1612**	**2,1**	**2,8**

Among women, the highest number of new cases was recorded in Constantine and Setif. The wilayas of Souk-Ahras, Batna, Bejaia and El Oued recorded high rates.

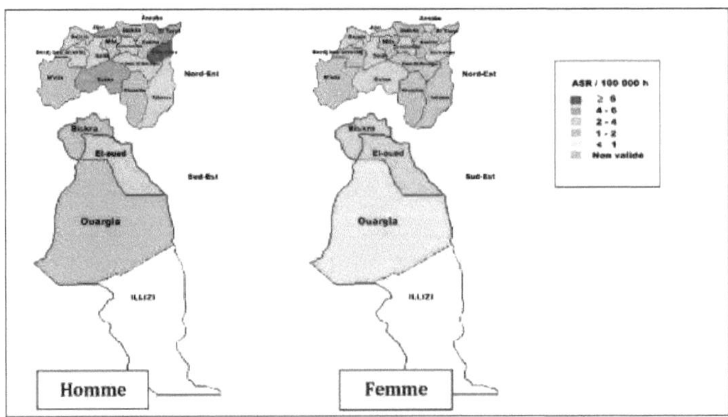

Figure 53. Mapping of pancreatic cancers, ESEA region 2014 - 2018.

3.4.5. Liver cancer

3.4.5.1. Incidence of liver cancer (ICD-10: C22) (East and South-East network), 2014-2018

Table 26: Crude, standardised, mean and rank incidence of liver cancer in both sexes (East and South East Network), 2014 - 2018.

Year	2014		2015		2016		2017		2018		Average	
Gender	H	F	H	F	H	F	H	F	H	F	H	F
Number of new case	99	64	98	87	125	79	147	116	164	157	**633**	**503**
Gross rate	1,2	0,8	1,2	1,1	1,5	1,0	1,7	1,4	1,9	1,8	**1,6**	**1,3**
Standardized rate	1, 7	1,2	1,7	1,5	2,2	1,4	2,4	2,1	2,6	2,6	**2,2**	**1,9**
% / other cancers	1,7	0,9	1,4	0,8	1,6	0,8	1,8	1,1	2,0	1,4	**1,7**	**1,0**

The estimated number of new cases of liver cancer between 2014 and 2018 is 1136, of which 58% are in men. Liver cancer accounts for only 5% of digestive cancers, of which it is the fifth most common cancer in men and women. The ratio of men to women is 1.26.

There has been a slight increase in the crude and standardised incidence rates since 2017, which are 1.7 and 2.4 for men and 1.4 and 2.1 per 100,000 inhabitants for women. Liver cancers have a very low frequency in both sexes (1.7% of male cancers and 1% of female cancers).

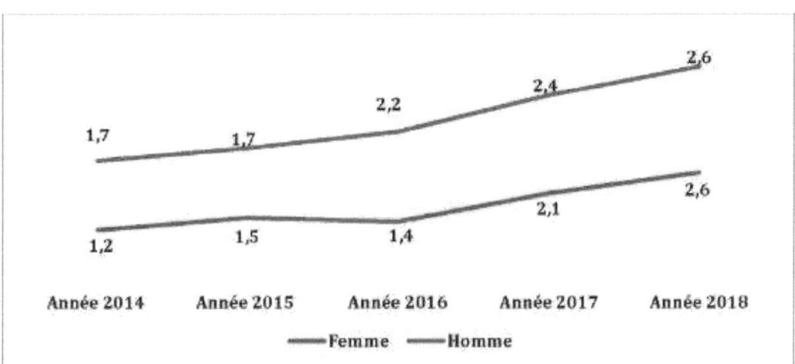

Figure 54. Trend in standardised incidence of liver cancer in both sexes, East and South-East region, 2014 - 2018.

For both sexes, the standardised incidence is gradually increasing. From 2014 to 2018, it increases from 1.7 to 2.6 and from 1.2 to 2.6 per 100,000 inhabitants respectively.

3.4.5.2. Variations in liver cancer incidence by age (East and South-East network), 2017

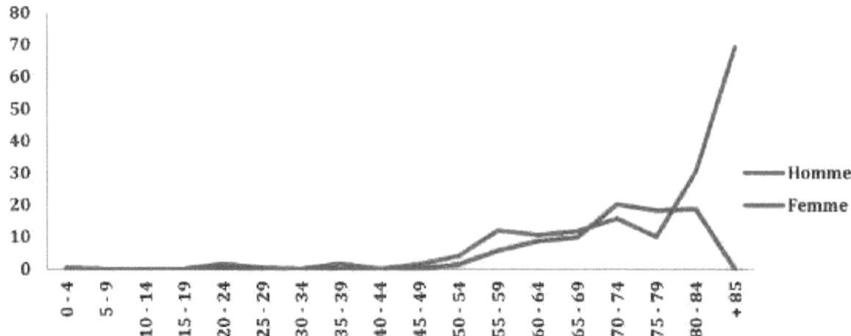

Figure 55. Distribution of standardised liver cancer rates by age and sex, ESEA region 2017.

In 2017, the median age at diagnosis is 63 years for men and 72 years for women. The cross-sectional curve of incidence rates according to age shows a marked progression of incidence rates from the age of 55 for both sexes, reaching a maximum value of 15.6 in men and 20.2 in women per 100,000 between the ages of 70 and 64, followed by a 2®me peak in men of 69.4 at over 80 years of age.

3.4.5.3. Geographical variations in the incidence of liver cancer

3.4.5.3.1. Standardised incidences of liver cancer from selected ESEA registries, 2017

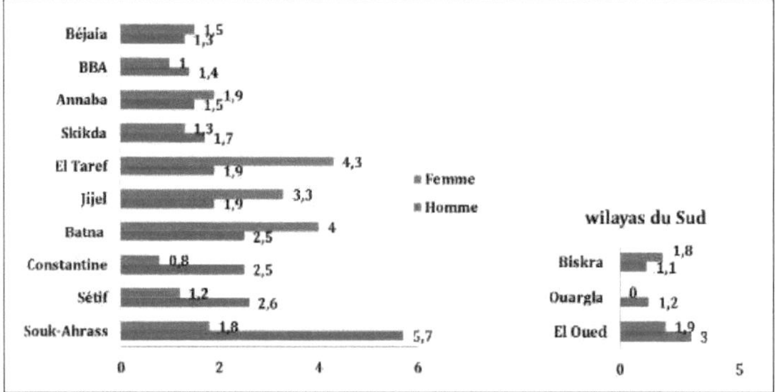

Figure 56. Comparison of standardised incidences of liver cancer in some registries of the East and South-East network, 2017.

In men, in 2017 the highest incidence of hepatic cancer was recorded in Souk-Ahras (5.7), El Oued (3.0) and Setif (2.5) BBA and Batna (2.5). In women, the wilayas most affected were Batna (4.0) and El Taref (4.3), while the other wilayas had an incidence of less than 2 per 100 000 inhabitants.

The Ouargla register does not record any cases of liver cancer in women.

The ratio of men to women varies in the different registers in the region.

3.4.5.3.2. Geographical variations in the mean incidence of liver cancer in both sexes.

Table 27. Distribution of the number of cases, mean crude and standardised incidence, of liver cancer according to the different registries of the Reseau Est and Sud- Est in men, 2014 - 2018.

Register	Total number of cases	Average gross rate*.	Average standardised rate
El Oued	34	2,7	5,1
Souk-Ahras	27	3,3	4,1
El Taref	12	2,3	3,6
Batna	63	1,8	2,9
Biskra	27	1,3	2,7
Annaba	39	2,4	2,6
Setif	55	1,4	2,0
Jijel	26	1,4	2,0
Bejaia	34	1,3	1,8
Tebessa	14	1,2	1,6
Constantine	32	1,2	1,5
BBA	13	0,8	1,0
Skikda	15	0,7	0,9
Ouargla	7	0,4	0,8
Oum El Bouaghi	10	0,7	0,7
East and South East Region	**461**	**1,6**	**2,2**

In men, it is the wilaya of Batna that recorded a significant number of cases of liver cancer (63 cases) during the period 2014 - 2018 followed by Setif, Annaba and El Oued.

The wilayas of Souk-Ahras, El Oued and El Taref had a higher average crude and standardised incidence than the region. The standardised average rates of Batna, Biskra, Annaba and Setif are close to those of the region.

The other wilayas recorded medium to low incidence rates.

Table 28. Distribution of the number of cases, mean crude and standardised incidence, of liver cancer according to the different registries of the Reseau Est and Sud- Est in women, 2014 - 2018.

Register	Total number of cases	Average gross rate*.	Average standardised rate
Batna	63	2,1	37
Souk-Ahras	23	2,8	3,5
Jijel	29	1,7	2,7
El Oued	18	1,5	2,5
El Taref	13	1,6	2,3
Tebessa	13	1,1	2,0
Annaba	26	1,8	1,9
Biskra	22	1,0	1,8
Oum el Bouaghi	19	1,3	1,6
Bejaia	24	1,0	1,3
BBA	17	0,9	1,3
Setif	38	0,9	1,2
Skikda	16	0,7	1,1
Constantine	22	0,8	0,8
Ouargla	2	0,1	0,2
East and South East Region	**409**	**1,3**	**1,9**

Among women, the highest number of new cases is recorded in Batna. The wilayas of Souk-Ahras, Batna, Jijel and El Oued recorded high rates.

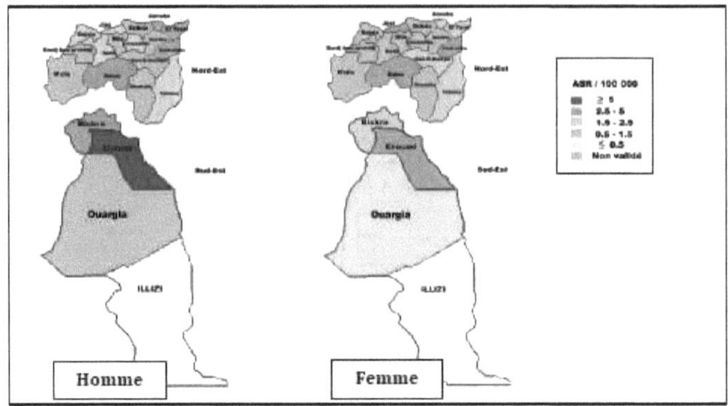

Figure 57. Mapping of liver cancers, ESEA region 2014 - 2018.

3.4.6. Cancer of the esophagus

3.4.6.1. Incidence of Resophageal Cancer (ICD-10: C22) (East and South East Network), 2014-2018

Table 29: Crude, standardised, mean and rank incidence of resophageal cancer in both sexes (East and South East Network), 2014 - 2018.

Year	**2014**		**2015**		**2016**		**2017**		**2018**	**Average**
Gender	**H**	**F**	**H**	**F**	**H**	**F**	**H**	**FH**	**FH**	**F**
Number of new case	47	26	47	45	77	54	69	29 74	47 **314**	**201**
Gross rate	0,6	0,3	0,6	0,6	0,9	0,7	0,8	0,4 0,8	0,6 **0,8**	**0,5**
Standardized rate	0,8	0,5	0,8	0,7	1,4	0,7	1,2	0,5 1,0	0,8 **1,1**	**0,7**
% / other cancers	0,9	0,4	0,7	0,5	1,0	0,6	0,8	0,3 0,9	0,4 **0,9**	**0,4**

The estimated number of new cases of resophageal cancer between 2014 and 2018 was 515, 60% of which were in men. [eme]It accounts for less than 3% of digestive cancers, and is the 6th most common cancer in men and women. It affects men 1.6 times more than women.

There has been a slight increase in incidence rates from 2014 to 2018.

In 2018, the crude and standardised rates were 0.8 and 1.0 per 100,000 for men and 0.6 and 0.8 per 100,000 for women respectively

C'est un cancer rare chez les deux sexes (0,9% chez l'homme et 0,4 chez la femme).

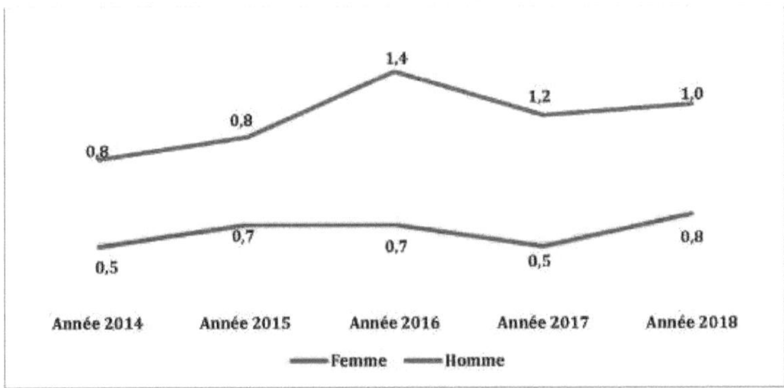

Figure 58. Trend in standardised incidence of resophageal cancer in both sexes, East and South-East region, 2014 - 2018.

The variation in standardised incidences of these cancers is not stable, fluctuating between 0.8 and 1.4 in men and 0.5 and 0.8 in women.

3.4.6.2. Age-specific variations in resophageal cancer incidence (East and South-East Network), 2017

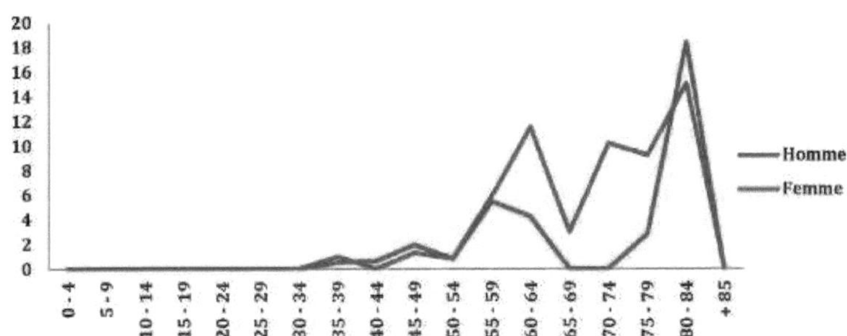

Figure 59. Distribution of standardised rates of resophageal cancer by age and sex, ESEA region 2017

In 2017, the median age at diagnosis was 62 years for both sexes. The cross-sectional curve of incidence rates according to age shows a marked progression of incidence rates from the age of 50 onwards in both sexes, reaching a maximum value of 11.5 per 100,000 in men and 5.44 in women between the ages of 55 and 59, followed by a 2®me peak of 15.0 in men and 18.4 in women between the ages of 80 and 84.

3.4.6.3. Geographical variations in the incidence of resophageal cancers

3.4.6.3.1. Standardised incidence of resophageal cancers in selected ESEA registries, 2017

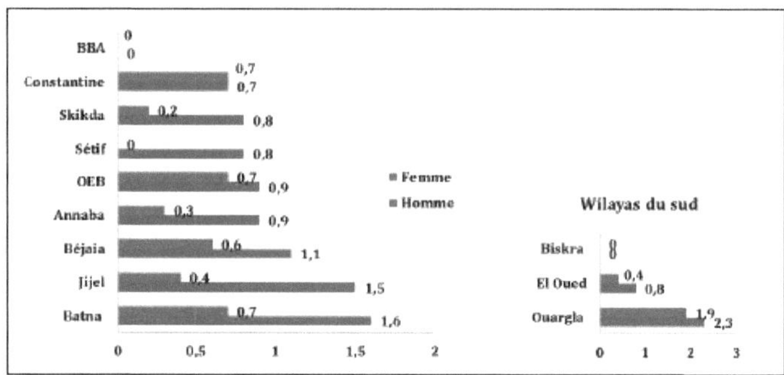

Figure 60: Comparison of standardised incidences of resophageal cancers in some registries of the East and South-East network, 2017.

In men, in 2017, the highest incidence of resophageal cancer was recorded in Ouargla (2.3), Batna (1.6) and Jijel (1.5). While in women, the wilayas most concerned are Ouargla (1.9), Batna and Constantine (0.7), the other wilayas had a lower incidence.

The BBA and Biskra registers did not record any cases of resophageal cancer.

The wilaya of Setif recorded 6 male cases.

The male predominance is confirmed in almost all wilayas (except for Constantine where the sex ratio = 1).

3.4.6.3.2. Geographical variations in the mean incidence of resophageal cancers in both sexes.

Tableau 30. Distribution of the number of cases, mean crude and standardised incidence, of resophageal cancer according to the different registries of the East and South-East Network in men, 2014 - 2018.

Register	Total number of cases	Average gross rate*.	Average standardised rate
El Oued	15	1,2	2,1
Jijel	15	0,9	1,6
Ouargla	13	0,8	1,5
Batna	26	0,8	1,4
Annaba	16	1,1	1,2
Souk-Ahras	5	0,6	0,9
Bejaia	18	0,6	0,8
Skikda	12	0,6	0,8
Setif	30	0,6	0,7
Biskra	5	0,2	0,6
El Taref	3	0,4	0,6
Oum El Bouaghi	7	0,5	0,5
BBA	5	0,3	0,4
Tebessa	4	0,3	0,4
Constantine	7	0,2	0,3

East and South-East Region	**198**	**0,8**	**1,1**

In men, the wilaya of Setif recorded the highest number of cases of resophageal cancer (30 cases) during the period 2014 - 2018, followed by Bejaia, Annaba and El Oued.
The wilayas of El Oued, Jijel, Annaba, Batna and Ouargla had a higher average crude and standardised incidence than those in the region. The other wilayas had medium to low incidence rates.

The wilaya of Constantine recorded only 6 cases during 2014 - 2018.

Tableau 31. Distribution of the number of cases, mean crude and standardised incidence, of resophageal cancer according to the different registries of the Reseau Est and Sud-Est in women, 2014 - 2018.

Register	Total number of cases	Average gross rate*.	Average standardised rate
El Oued	8	0,7	1,1
Annaba	13	0,9	0,9
Batna	20	0,6	0,9
Ouargla	12	0,7	0,8
Tebessa	6	0,5	0,7
BBA	7	0,4	0,6
Bejaia	11	0,5	0,5
Setif	15	0,4	0,5
El Taref	3	0,4	0,5
Souk-Ahras	4	0,5	0,5
Constantine	9	0,4	0,4
Biskra	6	0,2	0,3
Skikda	5	0,2	0,3
Oum El Bouaghi	4	0,3	0,3
Jijel	2	0,1	0,2
East and South-East Region	**138**	**0,5**	**0,7**

Among women, the highest number of new cases was recorded in Batna. The wilayas of El Oued, Batna and Annaba recorded high rates.

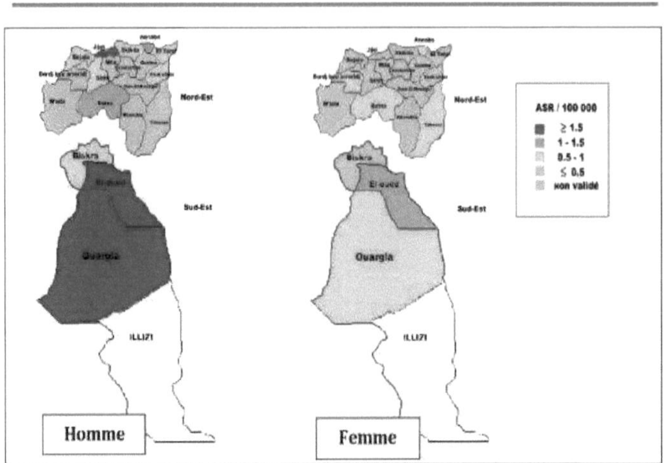

Figure 61. Mapping of resophageal cancers, ESEA region 2014 - 2018.

3.4.7. Graft bowel cancer

3.4.7.1. Incidence of Grele Bowel Cancer (ICD-10: C17) (East and South East Network), 2014-2018

Table 32: Crude, standardised, mean and rank incidence of graft bowel cancer in both sexes (East and South-East Network), 2014 - 2018.

Year	2014		2015		2016		2017		2018		Average	
Gender	H	F	H	F	H	F	H	F	H	F	H	F
Number of new case	52	12	57	38	64	54	67	64	60	50	**300**	**218**
Gross rate	0.6	0.2	0,7	0,5	0,8	0,7	0,8	0,8	0,7	0,6	**0,7**	**0,6**
Rate Standardise*	0,8	0,2	1,1	0,6	0,9	0,9	1,1	1,1	0,8	0,8	**1,0**	**0,8**
% / other cancers	0,9	0,2	0,8	0,3	0,6	0,5	0,8	0,6	0,7	0,4	**0,8**	**0,4**

The estimated number of new cases of transplanted bowel cancer between 2014 and 2018 was 518, 60% of which were in men. [me]It accounts for less than 3% of digestive cancers, and is the 6th most common cancer (same rank as resophageal cancer) in men and women. It affects men 1.4 times more than women.

In 2018, the crude and standardised rates were 0.7 and 0.8 for men and 0.6 and 0.8 per 100,000 inhabitants for women respectively. Small bowel cancer is one of the few cancers in both sexes (0.8% in men and 0.4 in women).

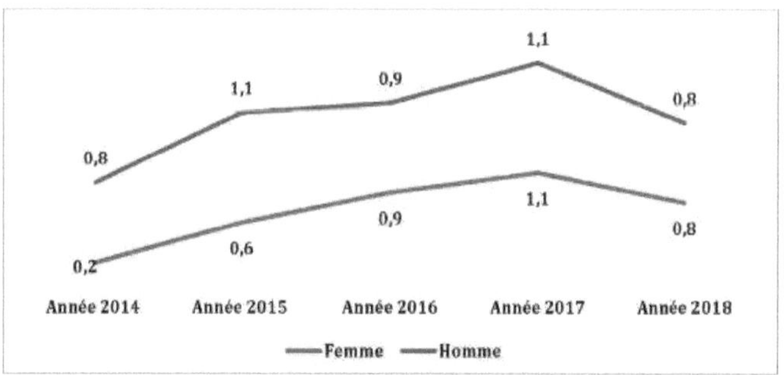

Figure 62. Trend in standardised incidence of grafted bowel cancer in both sexes, East and South-East region, 2014 - 2018.

In men, the standardised incidence is stable, while in women it is slightly increasing, from 0.2 in 2014 to 1.1 per 100 000 inhabitants in 2017.

3.4.7.2. Variations in the incidence of squamous bowel cancer by age (East and South-East Network), 2017 :

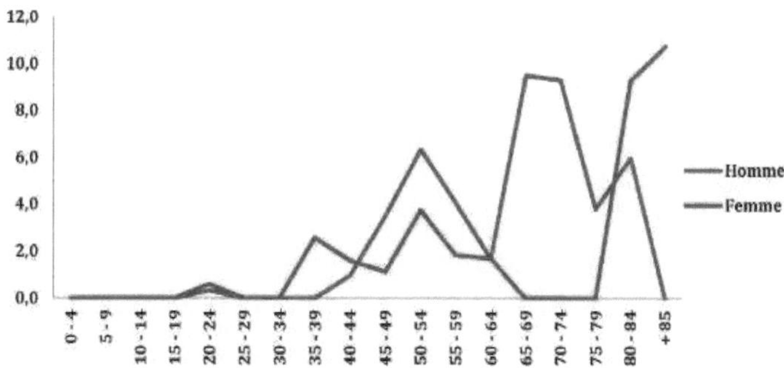

Figure 63. Distribution of standardised rates of graft bowel cancer by age and sex, ESEA region 2017.

The median age at diagnosis in 2017 was 57 for men and 52 for women. emeThe cross-sectional curve of incidence rates according to age shows a marked progression of incidence rates from the age of 35 in women and 50 in men, reaching a maximum value of 6.3 per 100,000 in men and 3.7 in women between the ages of 50 and 54, followed by a peak of 9.5 per 100,000 in men between the ages of 65 and 69 and 10.7 per 100,000 in women over 80.

3.4.7.3. Geographical variations in the incidence of squamous bowel cancer

Standardised incidence of bowel cancer in selected ESEA registries, 2017

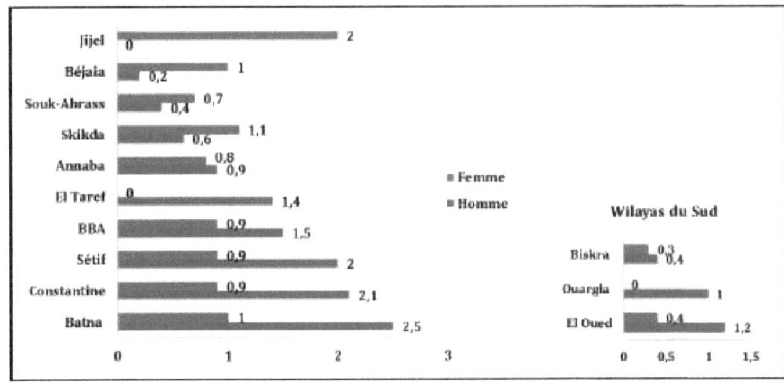

Figure 64. Comparison of standardised incidences of grafted bowel cancer from some registries in the East and South-East network, 2017.

In men, in 2017, the highest incidence of graft bowel cancer was recorded in Batna (2.5), Constantine (2.1), Setif (2.0) and BBA (1.5). While in women, the wilayas most concerned are Jijel (2.0), Skikda (0.7) and Bejaia, the other wilayas had a low incidence.

The relationship between men and women varies from one register to another.

3.4.7.3.1. Geographical variations in the mean incidence of graft bowel cancer in both sexes.

Table 33. Distribution of the number of cases, mean crude and standardised incidence of graft bowel cancer in the different registries of the East and South-East Network in men, 2014 - 2018.

Register	Total number of cases	Average gross rate*.	Average standardised rate
Annaba	20	1,4	1,5
Setif	33	0,8	1,2
Constantine	23	0,8	1,0
Ouargla	7	0,5	1,0
Bejaia	21	0,6	0,9
Jijel	9	0,5	0,9
Biskra	8	0,4	0,6
Batna	13	0,3	0,5
Oum el Bouaghi	5	0,3	0,5
BBA	5	0,3	0,5
El Taref	2	0,3	0,5
El Oued	4	0,3	0,5
Skikda	8	0,4	0,4
Souk-Ahras	2	0,2	0,3
Tebessa	2	0,2	0,3
East and South-East Region	**174**	**0,7**	**1,0**

In men, the wilaya of Setif recorded the highest number of cases of cancer of the small intestine (33 cases) during the period 2014 - 2018, followed by Constantine, Bejaia and Annaba.

The wilayas of Annaba and Setif had a higher average crude and standardised incidence than the region. Constantine, Ouargla, Jijel and Bejaia had a similar incidence.

The other wilayas recorded low incidence rates.

Table 34. Distribution of the number of cases, mean crude and standardised incidence, of grafted bowel cancer according to the different registries of the East and South-East Network in women, 2014 - 2018.

Register	Total number of cases	Average gross rate*.	Standardised rate medium*.
Jijel	12	0,8	1,5
Bejaia	21	1,0	1,2
El Taref	7	0,9	1,1
Annaba	12	0,8	0,9
Setif	21	0,6	0,8
Constantine	15	0,5	0,6
BBA	8	0,5	0,6
El Oued	4	0,3	0,5
Biskra	6	0,3	0,5
Batna	7	0,3	0,4
Skikda	6	0,3	0,4
Oum el Bouaghi	5	0,3	0,3
Tebessa	3	0,3	0,3
Souk-Ahras	1	0,1	0,2
Ouargla	1	0,1	0,1
East and South East Region	**142**	**0,6**	**0,8**

Among women, the highest number of new cases was recorded in Setif and Bejaia (21 cases). The wilayas of Jijel, Bejaia and El Taref recorded high rates.

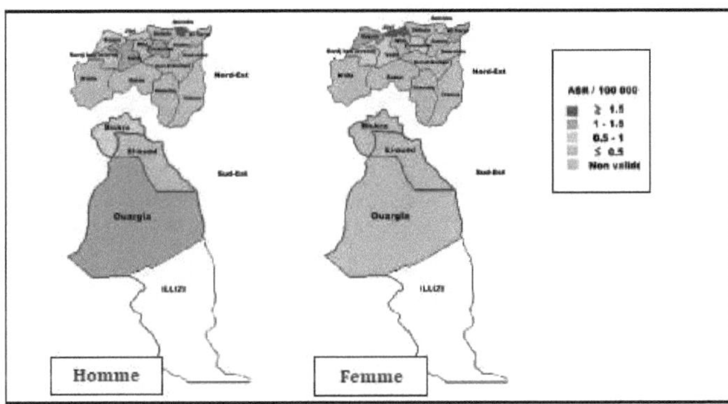

Figure 65. Mapping of bowel cancers in the ESEA region 2014 - 2018.

3.5. Digestive cancer incidence data by wilaya (East and South-East network), 2014 - 2018 :

3.5.1. Wilaya of Setif 2014 - 2018

3.5.1.1. Proportion of digestive cancers in both sexes in Setif ,2014 - 2018 :

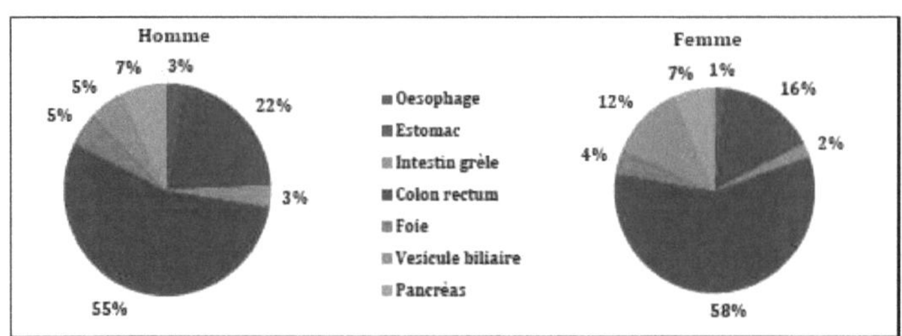

Figure 66. Distribution of digestive cancers in both sexes, Setif 2014 - 2018.

CRC is the most common cancer for both sexes with more than 50% followed by gastric cancer (22% for men and 16% for women).

In men, pancreatic cancer comes in 3eme position with 7%, while in women it is the cancer of the extrahepatic bile ducts and the VB with 12%. Cancers of the liver, resophagus and grafted intestine are less frequent in Setif.

3.5.1.2. Incidence of all digestive cancers in both sexes, Setif 2014-2018:

Table 35: Crude, standardised incidence and rank of all digestive cancers in Setif, 2014 - 2018 in both sexes.

Year	2014		2015		2016		2017		2018	
Gender	H	F	H	F	H	F	H	F	H	F
Number of cases	160	129	171	174	222	232	260	240	238	221
Gross rate	19,3	15,5	20,3	21,8	25,7	26,9	29,6	27,3	26,4	24,5
Standardized rate	26,2	20,3	28,2	29,1	39,7	37,9	41,0	34,9	36,6	31,0
% / other Cancers	25,9	15,8	23,7	17,3	25,9	17,3	29,7	17,4	25,8	14,7

There has been a marked increase in the number of new cases of digestive cancer, with 2047 cases recorded during this period, affecting both men and women. The average gross incidence was 24.6 in men and 24.8 in women, which corresponds to standardised rates of 36.4 and 33.2 respectively.

Digestive cancers represent more than 25% of male cancers and more than 15% of female cancers.

3.5.1.3. Incidence of all digestive cancers by age, Setif 2017:

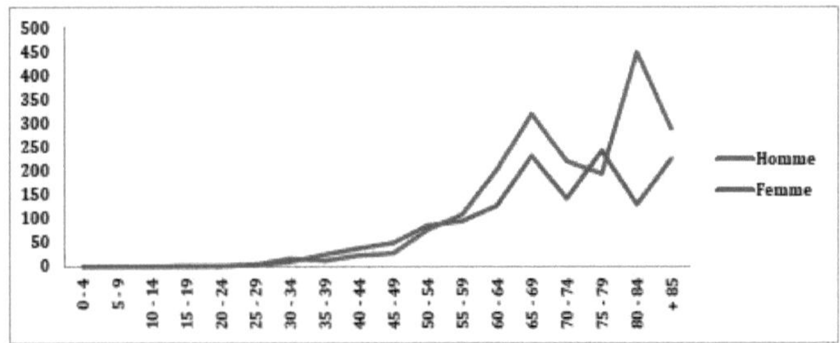

Figure 67. Distribution of standardised digestive cancer rates by sex and age group, Setif 2017.

90% of digestive cancers occur after the age of 40. The median age is 62 years for both sexes. The specific incidence rates increase progressively in both sexes to reach a maximum between 65 and 70 years of age (319.4 per 100,000 men and 231.3 per 100,000 women) and a second peak after 80 years of age in men.

3.5.1.4. Standardised incidence of digestive cancers by location in Setif, 2014 - 2018

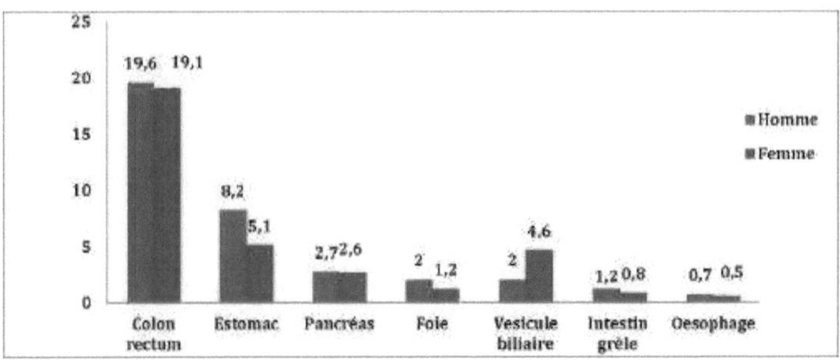

Figure 68. Comparison of mean standardised incidences of different digestive cancers by sex in Setif 2014 - 2018.

In both sexes, the highest incidence is for CRC and gastric cancer, with a male predominance for all digestive cancers except gallbladder cancer (4.6 in women and 2.0 per 100,000 population in men).

3.5.2. Wilaya of Batna 2014 - 2018

3.5.2.1. Proportion of digestive cancers in both sexes, Batna 2014 - 2018 :

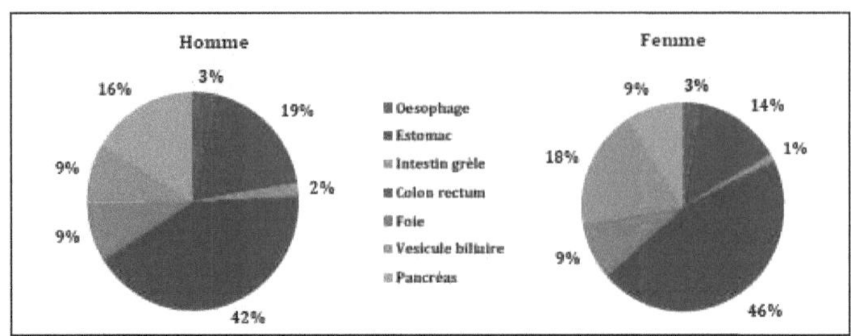

Figure 69. Distribution of digestive cancers in both sexes, Batna 2014 - 2018.

CRCs come in first place for both sexes, followed by gastric cancer (19% for men and 14% for women). In men, pancreatic cancer comes in third place with 16%, while in women it is extrahepatic bile duct and VB cancer with 18%.

Liver cancers in Batna represent 9% in both sexes, and those of the resophagus and the small intestine are less frequent.

3.5.2.2. Incidence of all digestive cancers in both sexes, Batna 2014-2018:

Table 36. Crude, standardised incidence and rank of all digestive cancers in Batna, 2014 - 2018 in both sexes.

Year	**2014**		**2015**		**2016**		**2017**		**2018**	
Gender	H	F	H	F	H	F	H	F	H	F
Number of cases	124	119	143	139	143	132	150	146	163	181
Gross rate	19,9	19,5	22,6	22,3	22,4	20,9	22,6	22,5	24,7	27,9
Standardized rate	30,5	29,3	34,3	34,1	35	31,7	39.9	38,7	37,9	42,5
% / other cancers	31,7	23,8	32,6	22,2	29	22,2	31,5	21,7	28,5	25,7

There has been a marked increase in the number of new cases of digestive cancer, with 1440 cases recorded during this period, affecting both men and women. The gross incidence in 2018 is 24.7 for men and 27.9 for women, which corresponds to standardised rates of 37.9 and 42.5 respectively.

Digestive cancers represent 30% of male cancers and more than 23% of female cancers.

3.5.2.3. Incidence of all digestive cancers according to age, Batna 2017:

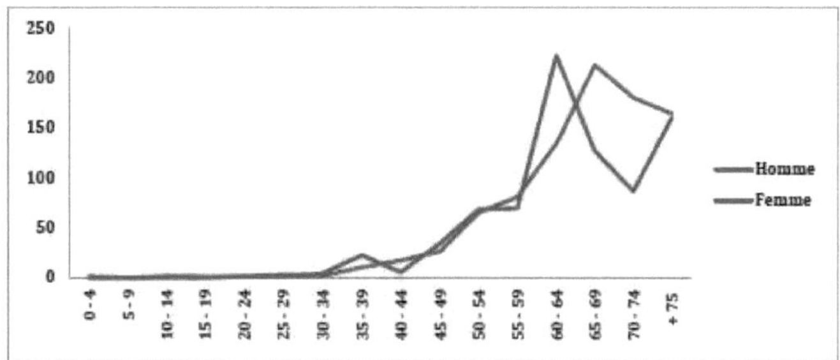

Figure 70. Distribution of standardised digestive cancer rates by age group and sex, Batna 2017. Digestive cancers are rare before the age of 40. The median age is 63 years for both sexes. The specific incidence rates increase progressively in both sexes to reach a maximum between 60-64 years of age in women (222.5 per 100,000 h) and between 65-69 years of age in men (213 per 100,000 h) and a second peak after 75 years of age in women.

3.5.2.4. Standardised incidence of digestive cancers by location in Batna, 2014-2018

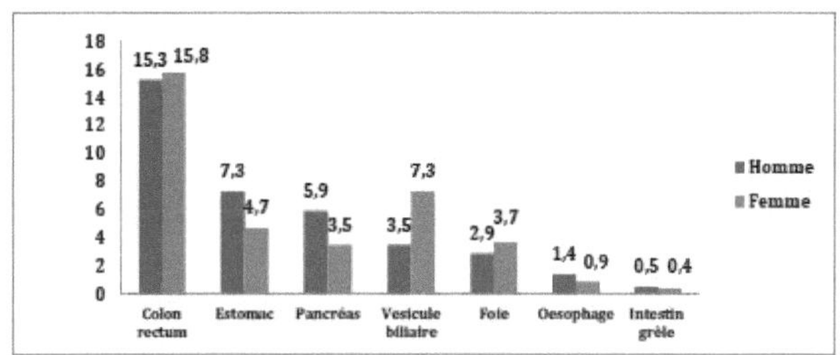

Figure 71. Comparison of mean standardised incidences of different digestive cancers by sex in Batna 2014 - 2018

In both sexes, the highest incidence is for CRC, gastric cancer and VB cancer. There is a female predominance for CRC and gallbladder cancer (7.3 in women and 3.5 per 100,000 population in men).

3.5.3. Wilaya of Constantine 2014 - 2018

3.5.3.1. Proportion of digestive cancers in both sexes Constantine, 2014 - 2018 :

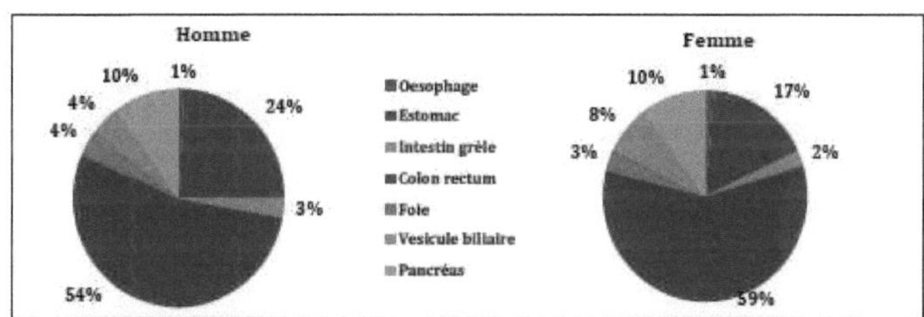

Figure 72. Distribution of digestive cancers in both sexes, Constantine 2014 - 2018.

CRCs represent more than half of all digestive cancers for both sexes, followed by gastric cancers

(24% for men and 17% for women). Pancreatic cancer comes in third place with 10%. emeHowever, in women, cancer of the extrahepatic bile ducts and VB comes in 5th position with only 8%. The other cancers are less frequent.

1.3.2 Incidence of all digestive cancers in both sexes, Constantine 2014-2018 :

Table 37. Crude, standardised incidence and rank of all digestive cancers in Constantine 2014 - 2018 in both sexes.

Annee20142015201620172018

Gender	H	F	H	F	H	F	H	F	H	F
Number of cases	129	114	148	106	132	118	176	172	197	162
Gross rate	24,5	21,5	27,3	20,1	24,9	22,4	32,8	32,0	30,8	25,7
Standardized rate	30,1	23,7	32,5	22,1	29,8	24,5	40,4	36,1	39,2	28,2
% / other Cancers	25,4	16,4	31,8	15,0	28,2	15,3	34,3	20,4	35,3	19,7

A clear increase in the number of new cases of digestive cancers has been noted since 2014, with 1454 cases recorded during this period, with a slight male predominance. The gross incidence in 2018 is 30.8 in men and 25.7 in women, which corresponds to standardised rates of 39.2 and 28.2 respectively.

Digestive cancers represent 30% of male cancers and more than 17% of female cancers.

3.5.3.3. Incidence of all digestive cancers according to age, Constantine 2017 :

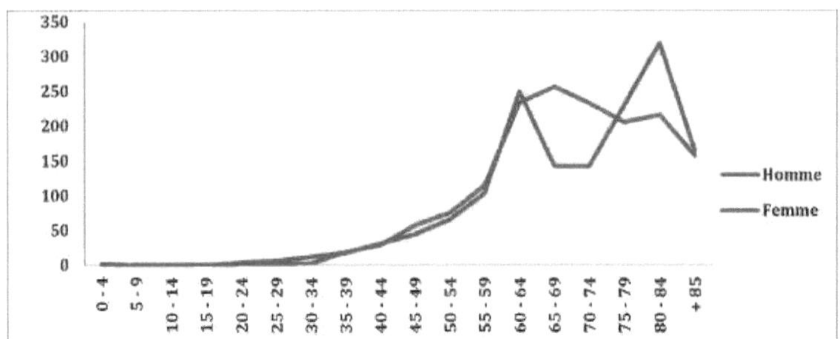

Figure 73. Distribution of standardised digestive cancer rates by age group and sex, Constantine 2017.

94% of digestive cancers occur after the age of 40. The median age is 67 years for both sexes.

The specific incidence rates increase progressively in both sexes, reaching a maximum between 60-64 with 248.9 per 100,000 in women and between 65-69 with 256.3 per 100,000 in men, and then a second peak after 80 years of age.

3.5.3.4 Standardised incidence of digestive cancers by location in Constantine, 2014 - 2018

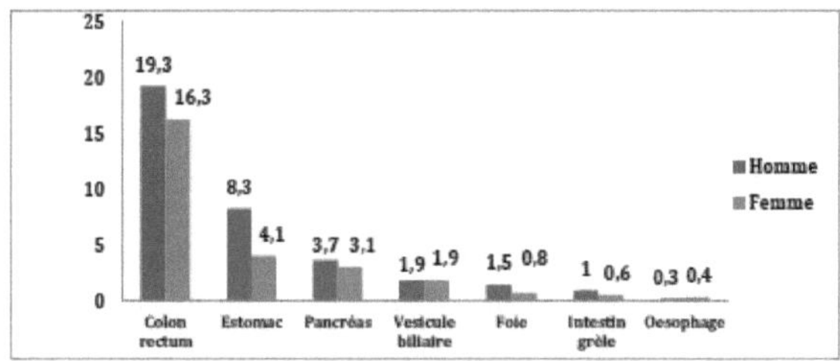

Figure 74. Comparison of mean standardised incidences of different digestive cancers by sex in Constantine 2014 - 2018.

In both sexes, the highest incidence is for CRC, gastric cancer and pancreatic cancer, with a male predominance. The Constantine registry recorded a low incidence of VB and HVLB cancer (1.9 per 100 000 inhabitants for both sexes).

3.5.4 Wilaya of Bejaia 2014 - 2018

3.5.4.1. Proportion of digestive cancers in both sexes, Bejaia 2014 - 2018 :

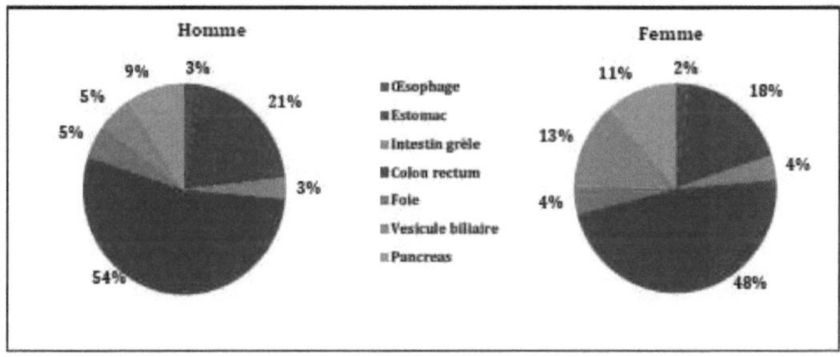

Figure 75. Distribution of digestive cancers in both sexes, Bejaia 2014 - 2018.

CRCs come first for both sexes with 54% in men and 48% in women, followed by gastric cancers with almost 20%.

In men, it is cancer of the pancreas which comes in third place with 9%, however, for women it is cancer of the extrahepatic bile ducts and the VB with 13%. The cancers of the liver, the resophagus and the grafted intestine are less frequent in this wilaya.

1.1.1.2. Incidence of all digestive cancers in both sexes, Bejaia 2014-2018:

Table 38: Crude, standardised incidence and rank of all digestive cancers in Bejaia, 2014 - 2018 in both sexes.

Year	2014		2015		2016		2017		2018	
Gender	H	F	H	F	H	F	H	F	H	F
Number of cases	105	72	152	133	160	142	119	172	126	104
Gross rate	21,7	15,5	31,3	28,7	32,7	30,4	24,2	22,5	25,4	22,0
Rate	25,9	17,8	41,0	30,7	41,1	32,1	30,0	25,6	31,5	25,0

Standardise* % / other Cancers	33,8	18,3	30,8	20,7	31,9	23,0	24,7	19,2	28,6	19,1

From 01 January 2014 to 31 December 2018, 1219 new cases of digestive cancer were recorded in Bejaia with a slight male predominance. There has been a rapid increase in crude and standardised incidence, reaching a maximum of 32.7 and 41.1 in men and 30.4 and 32.1 in women respectively in 2016, and then falling in 2018.
Digestive cancers represent 30% of male cancers and more than 20% of female cancers.

1.1.1.3. Incidence of all digestive cancers according to age, Bejaia 2017 :

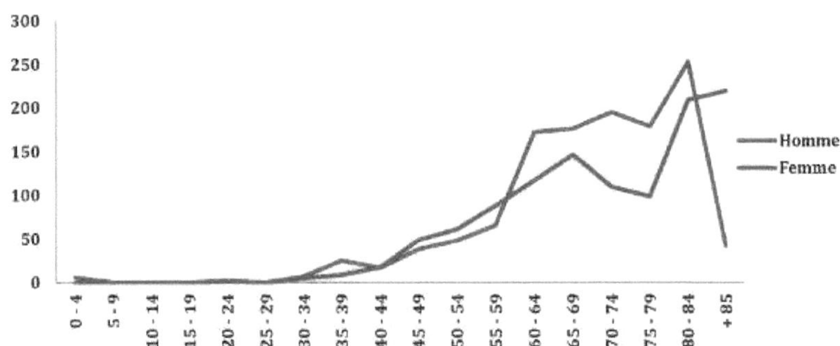

Figure 76. Distribution of standardised digestive cancer rates by age group and sex, Bejaia 2017.

Digestive cancers are rare before the age of 40. The median age is 63 years for both sexes.

The specific incidence rates increase progressively in both sexes, reaching a maximum between 65 - 69 with 146.1 per 100,000 in women and between 70 - 74 with 194.9 per 100,000 in men, followed by a second peak after the age of 80.

1.1.1.4. Standardised incidence of digestive cancers by location in Bejaia, 2014 - 2018

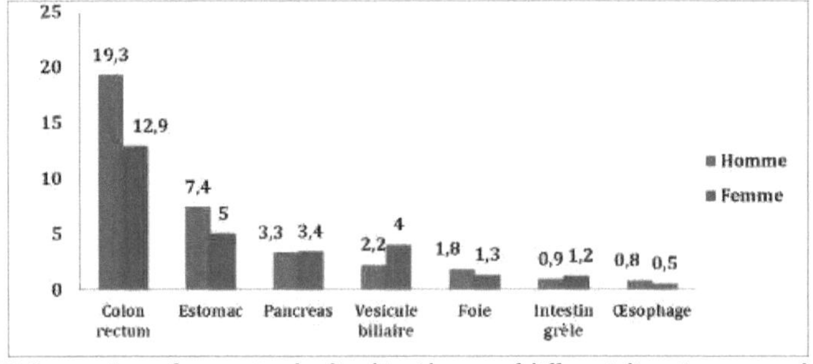

Figure 77. Comparison of mean standardised incidences of different digestive cancers by sex in Bejaia 2014 - 2018.

In men, the highest incidence is for CRC, gastric cancer and stomach cancer. emeIn women it is gallbladder cancer which comes in 3rd place (4 per 100,000 inhabitants in men).

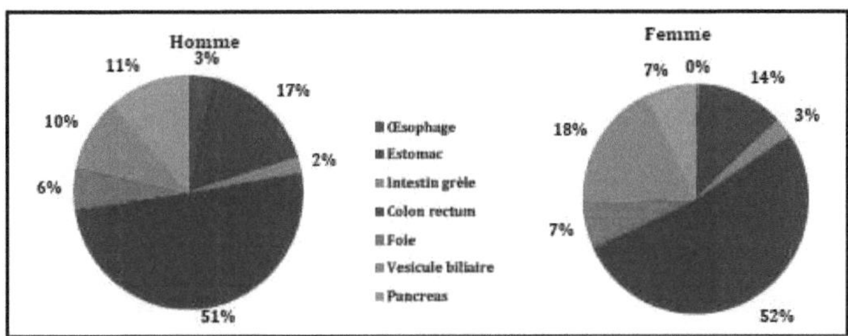

Figure 78. Répartition des cancers digestifs chez les deux sexes, Jijel 2014 – 2018.

3.5.5. Wilaya of Jijel 2014 - 2018

3.5.6. 1. Proportion of digestive cancers in both sexes, Jijel 2014 - 2018:Figure 78. Distribution of digestive cancers in both sexes, Jijel 2014 - 2018.

CRC is the most common cancer for both sexes with over 50% followed by gastric cancer (17% for men and 18% for women).

In men, it is pancreatic cancer that comes in third place with 11%, however, for women, it is cancer of the extrahepatic bile ducts and the VB with 18%. Liver cancers represent 6% for men and 7% for women. Cancers of the resophagus and of the small intestine are less frequent or even absent.

3.5.5.2. Incidence of all digestive cancers in both sexes, Jijel 2014-2018:

Table 39: Crude, standardised incidence and rank of all digestive cancers in Jijel, 2014 - 2018 in both sexes.

Year	**2014**		**2015**		**2016**		**2017**		**2018**	
Gender	**H**	**F**	**H**	**F**	**H**	**F**	**H**	**F**	**H**	**F**
Number of cases	57	64	73	83	78	91	93	96	139	114
Gross rate	15,8	17,8	20,0	23,0	20,8	25,1	24,5	25,8	36,2	30,2
Standardized rate	20,9	22,9	26,0	26,9	26,5	31,3	33,0	32,5	46,4	36,2
% / other cancers	25,4	20,4	26,6	21,1	23,3	24,5	21,7	19,1	30,1	24,6

888 cases of digestive cancer were recorded during this period, affecting both men and women. The gross and standardised incidence has increased rapidly in this wilaya, from 15.8 and 20.9 in men and 17.8 and 22.9 in women in 2014 to 36.2 and 46.4 and 30.2 and 36.9 respectively.

in 2014 to 36.2 and 46.4 and 30.2 and 36.2 respectively in 2018. Digestive cancers represent 25% of male cancers and 22% of female cancers.

3.5.5.3. Incidence of all digestive cancers according to age, Jijel 2017 :

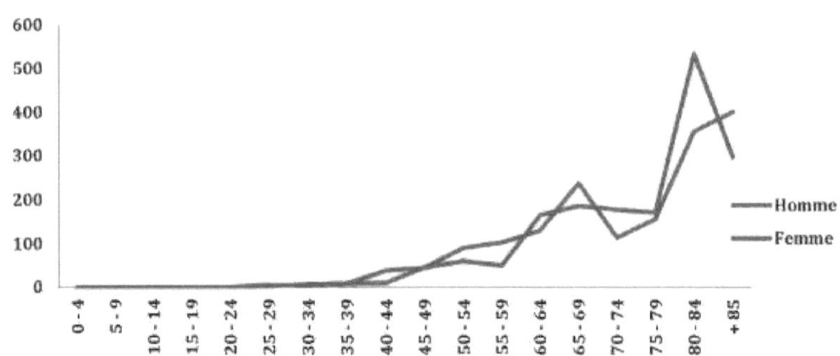

Figure 79. Distribution of standardised digestive cancer rates by age group and sex, Jijel 2017

Digestive cancers are rare before the age of 50. The median age is 67 years for both sexes.

The specific incidence rates increased progressively in both sexes, reaching a maximum between 65 and 69 years of age with 238 per 100,000 for men and 185.9 per 100,000 for women, and then a second peak after 80 years of age.

3.5.5.4. Standardised incidence of digestive cancers by location in Jijel, 2014 -2018

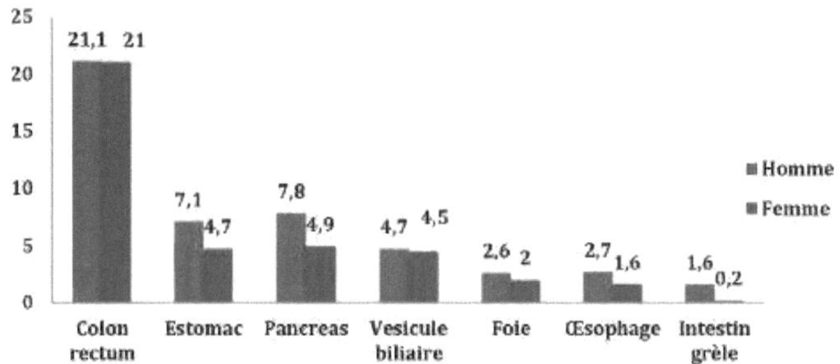

Figure 80. Comparison of mean standardised incidences of different digestive cancers by sex in Jijel 2014 - 2018.

In both sexes, the wilaya of Jijel records very high incidence rates of CRC and pancreatic cancer.

3.5.6 Wilaya of Annaba 2014 - 2018 :

3.5.6.1. Proportion of digestive cancers in both sexes, Annaba 2014 - 2018 :

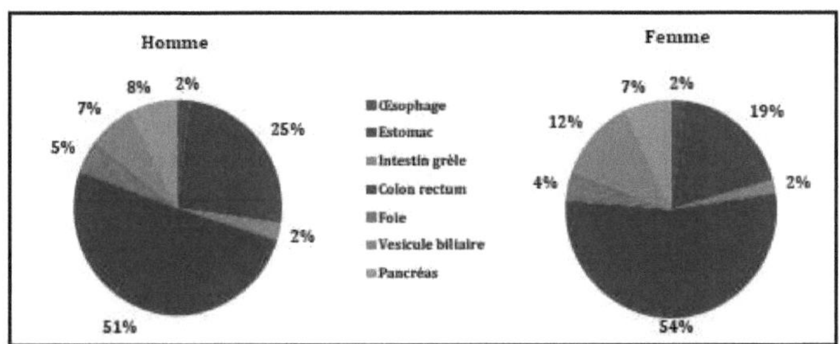

Figure 81. Répartition des cancers digestifs chez les deux sexes, Annaba 2014 - 2018.

Distribution of digestive cancers in both sexes, Annaba 2014 - 2018.

CRC is the most common cancer for both sexes with over 50% followed by gastric cancer (25% for men and 19% for women).

In men, cancer of the pancreas comes in third place with 8%, and in women it is cancer of the extrahepatic bile ducts and VB with 12%. Cancers of the liver, resophagus and grafted intestine are less frequent in Annaba.

1.1.1.2. Incidence of all digestive cancers in both sexes, Annaba 2014-2018:

Table 40: Crude, standardised incidence and rank of all digestive cancers in Annaba, 2014 - 2018 in both sexes.

Year	2014		2015		2016		2017		2018	
Gender	H	F	H	F	H	F	H	F	H	F
Number of case	51	47	153	143	214	164	181	130	195	138
Gross rate	15,1	14,0	43,8	41,4	59,4	46,0	50,2	36,2	54,1	38,5
Standardised*	17,2	16.0	49,8	44,6	66,8	51,3	55,2	39,6	61,6	43,2
rate % / other cancers	17,2	14,5	23,8	22,2	32,3	20,7	31,2	18,6	33,4	18,4

1456 new cases were recorded during this period, affecting 1.3 times more men than women. The wilaya of Annaba recorded the highest crude or standardised incidence rates in this region, reaching respectively, in 2016,

59.4 and 66.8 in men and 46.0 and 51.3 in women. Digestive cancers represent 28% of male cancers and 19% of female cancers.

1.1.1.3. Incidence of all digestive cancers according to age, Annaba 2017 :

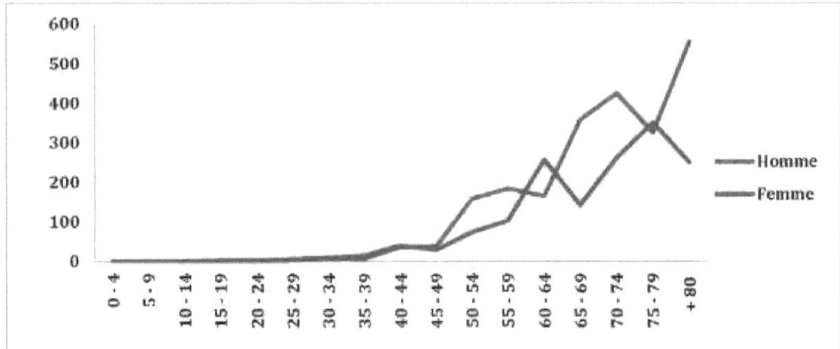

Figure 82. Distribution of standardised digestive cancer rates by age group and sex, Annaba 2017

The median age is 63 years for both sexes. The specific incidence rates increase for both sexes from the age of 50 onwards, reaching a maximum between 55 - 59 years with 183.3 per 100,000 in men and between 60 - 64 years with 256.2 per 100,000 in women, and a second peak after 70 years.

1.1.1.4. Standardised incidence of digestive cancers by location in Annaba, 2014 - 2018

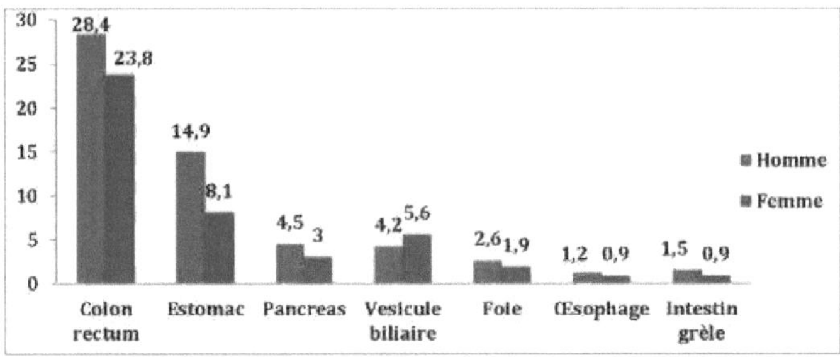

Figure 83. Comparison of mean standardised incidences of different digestive cancers by sex in Annaba 2014 - 2018.

In both sexes, this wilaya records very high rates of CRC and stomach cancer, which is different from other registers.

3.5.7. Wilaya of BBA 2015 - 2018

3.5.7.1. Proportion of digestive cancers in both sexes, BBA 2014 - 2018 :

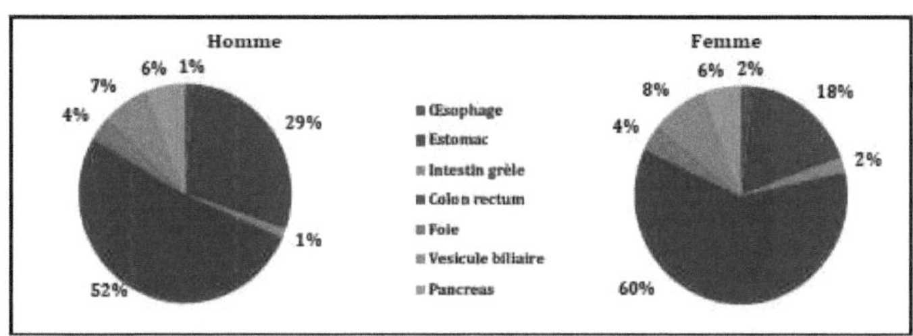

Figure 84. Distribution of digestive cancers in both sexes, BBA 2014 - 2018.

CRCs occupy the first position for both sexes with 52% in men and 60% in women followed by gastric cancers (22% for men and 16% for women). Other digestive cancers have low proportions between 2% and 8%.

3.5.7.2. Incidence of all digestive cancers in both sexes, BBA 2014-2018:

Table 41: Crude, standardised incidence and rank of all digestive cancers in BBA, 2014 - 2018 in both sexes.

Year	2014		2015		2016		2017		2018	
Gender	H	F	H	F	H		FH	F	H	F
Number of cases	71	81	58	48	59		5990	103	119	129
Gross rate	20,3	24,3	16,4	14,1	16,5	17,2	24,9	29,6	32,8	37,0
Rate Standardise*	28,1	32,9	22,7	20,7	24,2	23,2	36,4	37,8	45,4	50,3
% / other cancers	28,9	23,2	34,8	17,6	25.5	17,6	27,1	21,7	27,2	19,1

In 2018, there was a clear increase in the number of new cases of digestive cancers, with a significant increase in crude incidence of 32.8 in men and 37.0 in women, corresponding to standardised rates of 45.4 and 50.3.

Digestive cancers represent more than 29% of male cancers and more than 20% of female cancers.

3.5.7.3. Incidence of all digestive cancers by age, BBA 2017 :

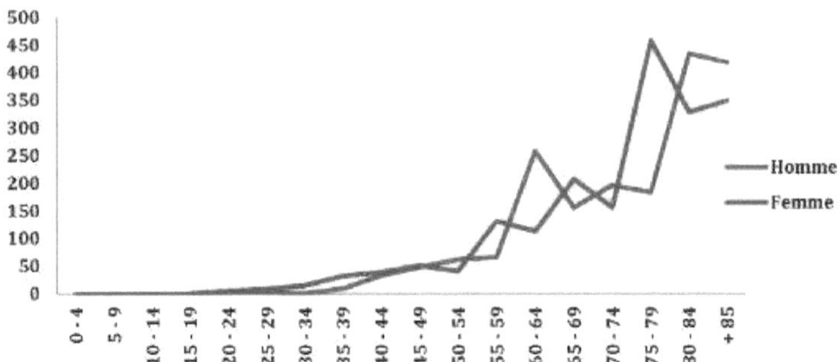

Figure 85. Distribution of standardised digestive cancer rates by age group and sex, BBA 2017.

The median age is 62 years for both sexes.

The specific incidence rates increase in both sexes from the age of 40 onwards, reaching a maximum between 60-64 years of age with 257.6 per 100,000 in men and between 65-69 years of age with 206.8 per 100,000 in women, followed by a second peak after the age of 75.

3.5.7.4. Standardised incidence of digestive cancers by location in BBA, 2014 -2018

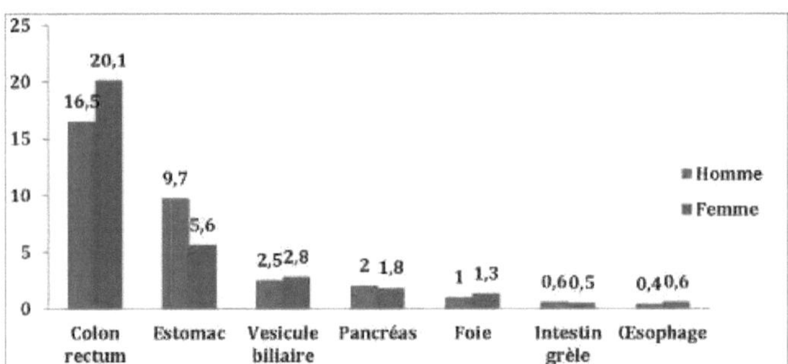

Figure 86. Comparison of mean standardised incidences of different digestive cancers by sex in BBA 2014 - 2018.

In both sexes, the highest incidence is for CRC with a female predominance (16.5 in men and 20.1 in women), followed by stomach cancer (9.7 per 100 000 men).

3.5.8. Wilaya of Biskra 2014 - 2018

3.5.8.1. Proportion of digestive cancers in both sexes, Biskra 2014 - 2018:

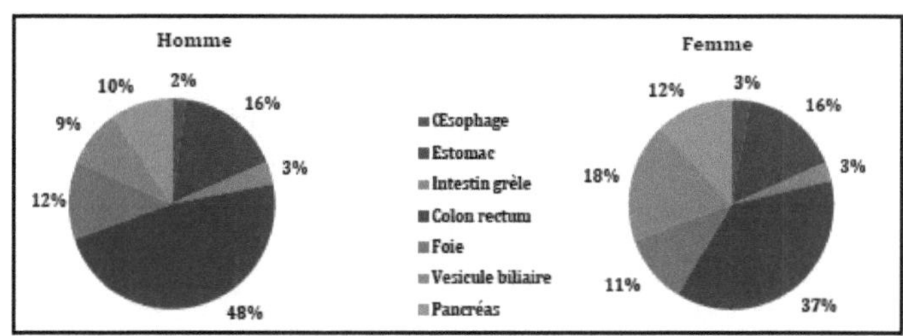

CRC takes the first position for both sexes but with less than 50% followed by gastric cancer in men and VB cancer in women. In men, liver cancer is in 3eme position with 12%, similarly for women, it is stomach cancer with 16%.

3.5.8.2 Incidence of all digestive cancers in both sexes, Biskra 2014-2018 :

Table 42: Crude, standardised incidence and rank of all digestive cancers in Biskra, 2014 - 2018 in both sexes.

Year	2014		2015		2016		2017		2018	
Gender	H	F	H	F	H	F	H	F	H	F
Number of cases	21	23	51	43	40	36	39	46	76	58
Gross rate	4,8	5,6	11,5	10.2	8,8	8,3	8,3	10,3	16,3	12,4
Rate Standardise*	7,1	7,5	18,4	15,4	13,9	13,3	14,2	15,5	42,1	28,3
% / other cancers	21	10,5	25,1	14,5	33,8	14,3	20,9	14,6	30,4	14,8

In 2018, there was a clear increase in the number of new cases of digestive cancers, especially in men. The gross incidence increased by 16.3 in men and 12.4 in women, which corresponds to standardised rates of 42.1 in men and 28.3 in women.

Digestive cancers represent 26% of male cancers and more than 14% of female cancers.

3.5.8.3 Standardised incidence of digestive cancers by location in Biskra, 2014 -2018

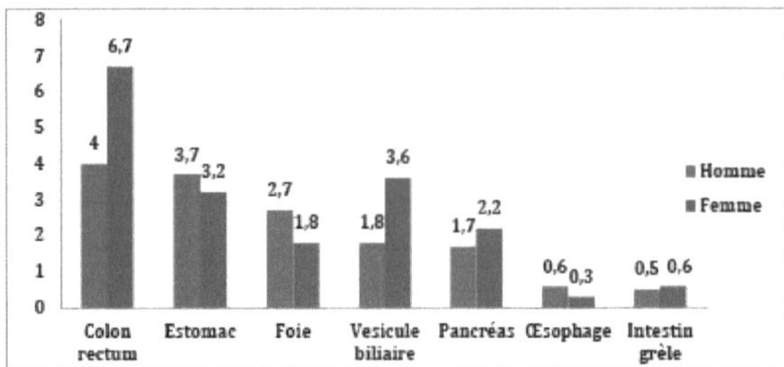

Figure 88. Comparison of mean standardised incidences of different digestive cancers by sex in Biskra 2014 - 2018.

In Biskra and according to the registry data, the incidence of CRC is low and it is diagnosed more in women than in men, however, VB cancer is present with an incidence of 3.6 per 100 000 women.

3.5.9. Wilaya of Ouargla 2014 - 2015

3.5.9.1 Proportion of digestive cancers in both sexes, Ouargla 2014 - 2018 :

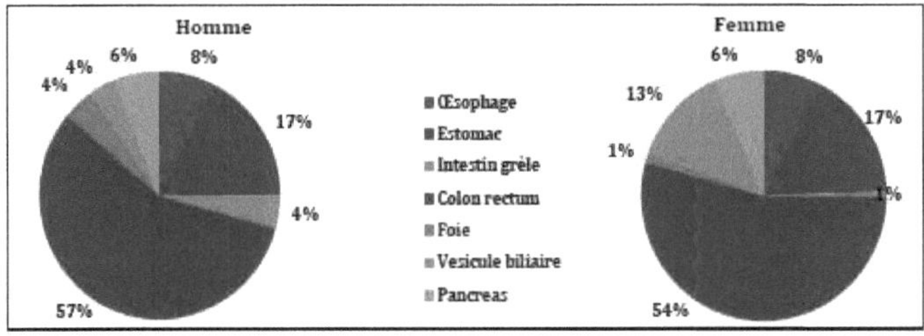

Figure 89. Distribution of digestive cancers in both sexes, Ouargla 2014 - 2018.

CRC is in first place for both sexes with more than 50% followed by gastric cancer (17%).

In men, cancer of the resophagus comes in third place with 8%, while in women it is cancer of the extrahepatic bile ducts and the VB with 13%.

3.5.9.2 Incidence of all digestive cancers in both sexes, Ouargla 2014-2018 :

Table 43: Crude, standardised incidence and rank of all digestive cancers in Ouargla, 2014 - 2018 in both sexes.

Year		2014		2015	2016		2017	2018
Gender	H	F	H	F	H	FH	FH	F
Number of cases	21	20	36	20	48	4528	3234	38
Gross rate	6,5	6,4	10,8	6,3	14,3	19,98,3	9,79,8	16,1

Rate Standardise*	10,5	11,8	19,7	10,8	24,4	22,6	13,6	18,4	11,1	21,9
% / other cancers	26,3	11,6	22	10	29,6	19,9	21,4	17	30,6	21,5

The number of new cases of digestive cancer remains low and stable in this wilaya. The gross and standardised incidence fluctuates from year to year.

3.5.9.3. Standardised incidence of digestive cancers by location in Ouargla, 2014 -2018

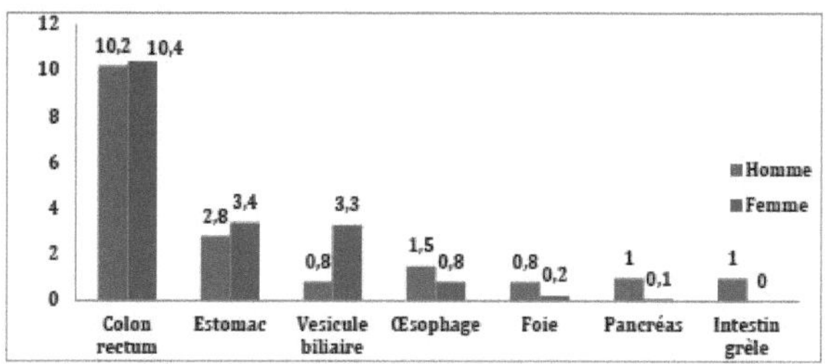

Figure 90. Comparison of mean standardised incidences of different digestive cancers by sex in Ouargla 2014 - 2018.

In Ouargla and according to the registry data the incidence of CRC is moderately low, however, VB cancer is present with an incidence of 3.6 per 100 000 women.

3.5.10. Wilaya of El Taref 2015 - 2018

3.5.10.1. Proportion of digestive cancers in both sexes, El Taref 2015 - 2018 :

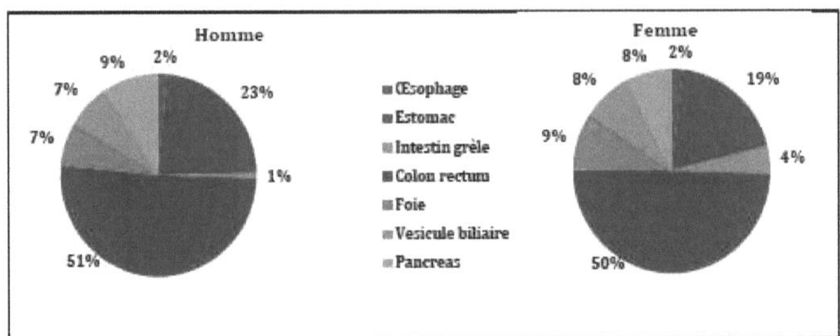

Figure 91. Répartition des cancers digestifs chez les deux sexes, El Taref 2015 - 2018.

Figure 91. Distribution of digestive cancers in both sexes, El Taref 2015 - 2018.

CRCs are in first place for both sexes with 50%, followed by gastric cancers (23% for men and 19% for women).

Pancreatic cancer with 9%, in men and liver cancer with 12%, in women, are in the 3eme position. Cancer of the resophagus and of the small intestine are less frequent.

3.5.10.1. Incidence of all digestive cancers in both sexes, El Taref 2016-2018:

Table 44: Crude, standardised and rank incidence of all digestive cancers in El Taref, 2016 - 2018 in both sexes.

Year	2016		2017		2018	
Gender	H	F	H	F	H	F
Number of cases	65	48	84	65	65	50
Gross rate	29,0	21,4	37,1	24,7	28,3	21,7
Rate Standardise*	35,4	25,5	48,6	31,3	37,9	26,8
% / other cancers	23	20,5	37,5	25,7	32,1	17,3

From 01 January 2016 to 31 December 2018, 377 new cases of digestive cancer were recorded in Taref with a slight male predominance. There has been a rapid increase in the crude and standardised incidence, reaching a maximum of

37.1 and 48.6 in men and 24.7 and 31.3 in women in 2017, and then declined significantly in 2018. Digestive cancers represent 30% of male cancers and 20% of female cancers.

3.5.10.3 Incidence of all digestive cancers by age, El Taref 2017 :

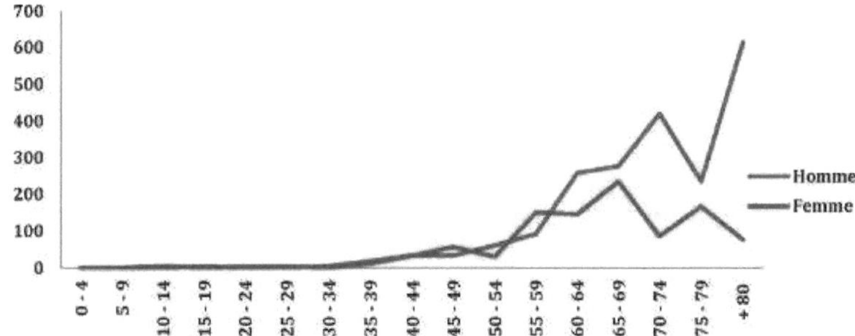

Figure 92. Distribution of standardised digestive cancer rates by age group and sex, El Taref 2017.

Digestive cancers are rare before the age of 50. The median age is 67 years for both sexes. The specific incidence rates increase progressively in both sexes to reach a maximum between 65-69 years of age in women (234.7 per 100,000) and between 70-74 years of age in men (420.4 per 100,000) and then a second peak after 75 years of age.

3.5.10.4 Standardised incidence of digestive cancers by location in El Taref 2016 -2018

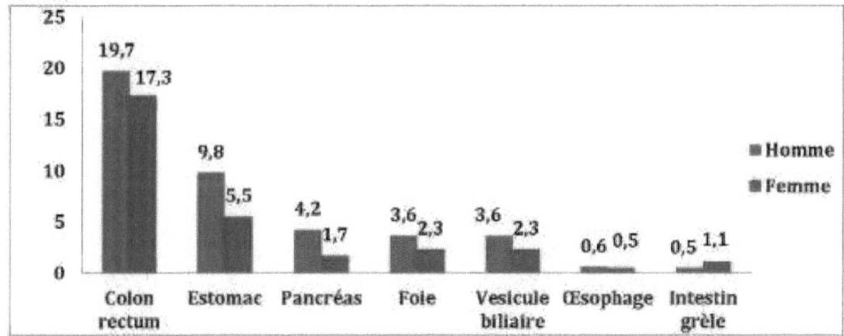

Figure 93. Comparison of mean standardised incidences of different digestive cancers by sex in El Taref 2016 - 2018.

In both sexes, the highest incidence is for CRC and gastric cancer, however liver cancer is present with a moderately high incidence in both sexes (3.6 in men and 2.3 in women).

3.5.11. Wilaya of Skikda 2015 - 2018

3.5.11.1. Proportion of digestive cancers in both sexes, Skikda 2015 - 2018 :

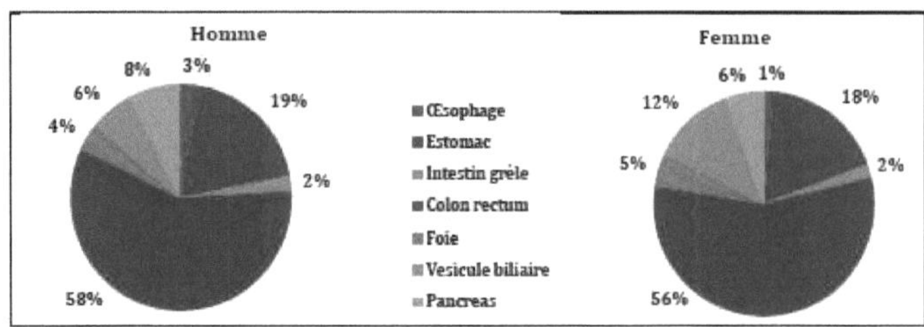

Figure 94. Distribution of digestive cancers in both sexes, Skikda 2015 - 2018.

CRC is the most common digestive cancer in both sexes with over 50%, followed by gastric cancer (19% for men and 18% for women).

In men, pancreatic cancer comes in third place with 8%, and in women, VB cancer with 12%.

3.5.11.2. Incidence of all digestive cancers in both sexes, Skikda 2015-2018:

Table 45: Crude, standardised incidence and rank of all digestive cancers in Skikda, 2015 - 2018 in both sexes.

Year	**2015**		**2016**		**2017**		**2018**	
Gender	H	F	H		FH	F	H	F
Number of cases	59	48	80	80	137	117	115	95
Gross rate	11,6	9,6	16	16,1	25,7	22,4	21,3	17,8
Rate Standardise*	14,9	9,6	20,6	20,1	32,5	28,7	26,4	21,7
% / other cancers	27,2	17,1	28,2	19,6	36,8	22,8	35,5	19,8

There has been a marked increase in the number of new cases of digestive cancers per year with a slight male predominance.

There has also been a rapid increase in crude and standardised incidence, reaching a maximum of 27.7 and 32.5 for men and 22.4 and 28.7 for women respectively in 2017, with these incidences falling in 2018.

3.5.11.3. Incidence of all digestive cancers according to age, Skikda 2017 :

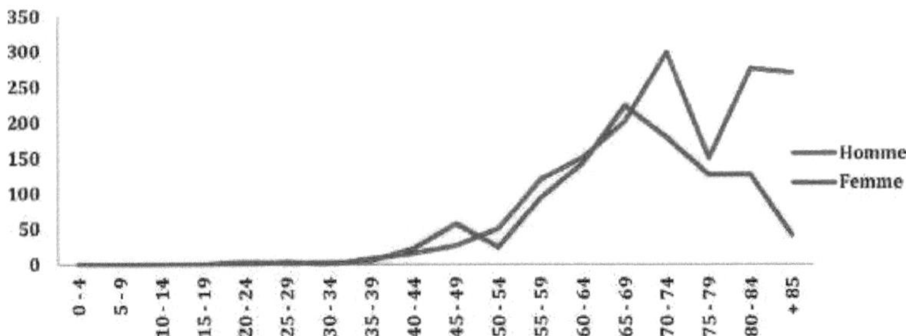

Figure 95. Distribution of standardised digestive cancer rates by age group and sex, Skikda 2017.

Digestive cancers were rare before the age of 40. The median age is 67 years for both sexes. The specific incidence rates increase progressively in both sexes to reach a maximum between 65-69 years of age in women (223.8 per 100,000) and between 70-74 years of age in men (298.6 per 100,000) and a second peak after 80 years of age in men.

3.5.11.4. Standardised incidence of digestive cancers by location in Skikda, 2015 - 2018

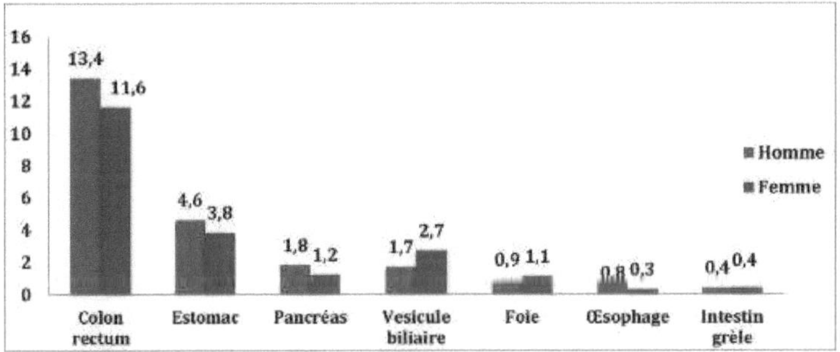

Figure 96. Comparison of mean standardised incidences of different digestive cancers by sex in Skikda 2015 - 2018.

According to the data of the register of this wilaya, the incidence of the various digestive cancers is moderately low, the highest being CRC.

3.5. 12. EPO Wilaya 2015 - 2018

3.5.12. 1. proportion of digestive cancers in both sexes, EPO 2015 - 2018 :

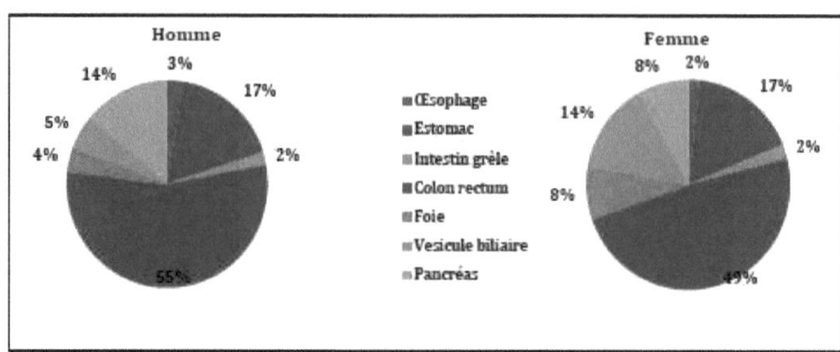

Figure 97. Distribution of digestive cancers in both sexes, EPO 2015 - 2018.

CRCs occupy the first position for both sexes with 55% in men and 49% in women, followed by gastric cancer (17%). In men, pancreatic cancer comes in 3eme position with 14%, and in women, VB cancer with 14%. Liver cancer represents 8% in women.

3.5.12.2 Incidence of all digestive cancers in both sexes, EPO 2015-2018 :

Table 46: Crude, standardised incidence and rank of all digestive cancers in EPO, 2015 - 2018 in both sexes.

Year	**2015**		**2016**		**2017**		**2018**	
Gender	H	F	H	F	H	F	H	F
Number of cases	57	46	39	32	62	75	106	81
Gross rate	15,1	12,8	9,9	8,4	16,4	19,8	27,6	21,2
Rate Standardise*	20,5	15,3	11,9	9,4	19,7	21,9	33,5	25,2
% / other cancers	29,2	15,3	23,1	12,1	36,4	21,9	34,2	19,0

The number of new cases of digestive cancers registered per year is increasing, with a slight male predominance. The crude incidence and standardised incidence are gradually increasing to reach a maximum of 27.6 and 33.5 in men and 21.2 and 25.2 in women respectively in 2018.

3.5.12.3 Standardised incidence of digestive cancers by location in EPO, 2015 -2018

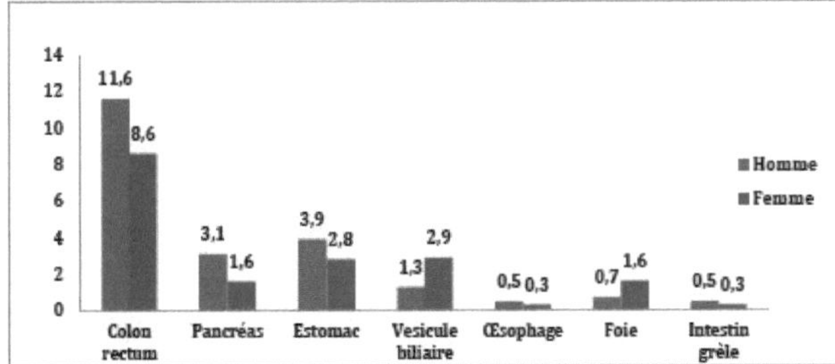

Figure 98. Comparison of average standardised incidences of different digestive cancers by sex in EPO 2015 - 2018

According to the data of the register of this wilaya, the incidence of the various digestive cancers is moderately low, the highest being that of CRC followed by that of the pancreas in men (3.1 per 100 000 inhabitants).

3.5.13. Wilaya of Souk-Ahras 2016 - 2018

3.5.13. 1. proportion of digestive cancers in both sexes, Souk-Ahras 2016 - 2018 :

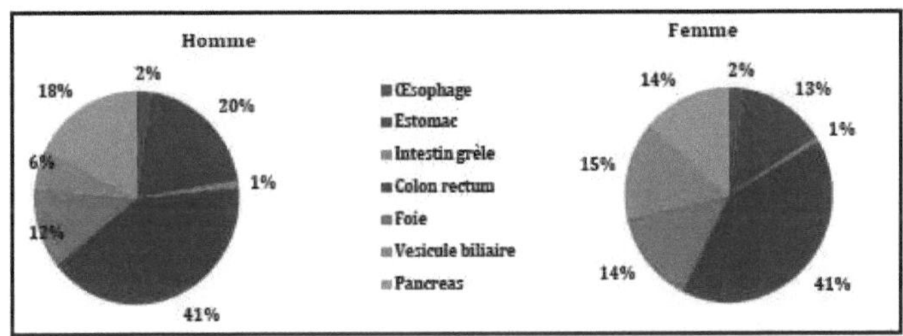

Figure 99. Distribution of digestive cancers in both sexes, Souk-Ahras 2016 - 2018.

Souk-Ahras, like all the wilayas, CRC is in first position for both sexes with 41%, followed by gastric cancer in men with 20% and VB in women with 15%.

In men, pancreatic cancer is in third place with 18%, followed by liver cancer, and in women with 14% for both locations. Cancer of the resophagus and of the small intestine are less frequent.

3.5.13.2. Incidence of all digestive cancers in both sexes, Souk-Ahras 2016-2018:

Table 47: Crude, standardised and rank incidence of all digestive cancers in Souk-Ahras, 2016 - 2018 in both sexes.

Year	2016		2017		2018	
Gender	H	F	H	F	H	F
Number of cases	53	41	73	50	92	71
Gross rate	21,8	16,4	28,5	19,5	35,3	27,1
Rate	26,9	18,7	35,2	23,0	44,7	34,4

Standardise* % / other cancers	21,8	16,5	28,1	15,4	30,0	17,6

The number of new cases of digestive cancers per year is increasing with a slight male predominance. There has been a remarkable increase in the standardised incidence in 2018, 44.7 in men and 34.4 in women.

3.5.13.3. Incidence of all digestive cancers according to age, Souk-Ahras 2017:

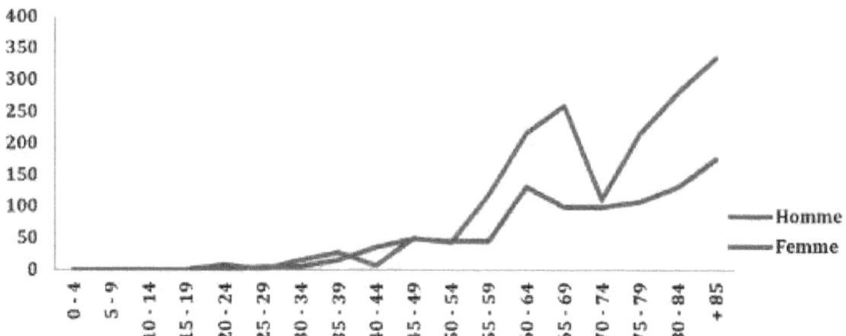

Figure 100: Distribution of standardised digestive cancer rates by age group and sex, Souk-Ahras 2017.

Digestive cancers are rare before the age of 40. The median age is 67 years for both sexes. The specific incidence rates increase progressively in both sexes to reach a maximum between 60-64 years of age in women (130.2 per 100,000) and between 65-69 years of age in men (258.7 per 100,000) and a second peak after 80.

3.5.13.4. Standardised incidence of digestive cancers by location in Souk-Ahras, 2016 -2018

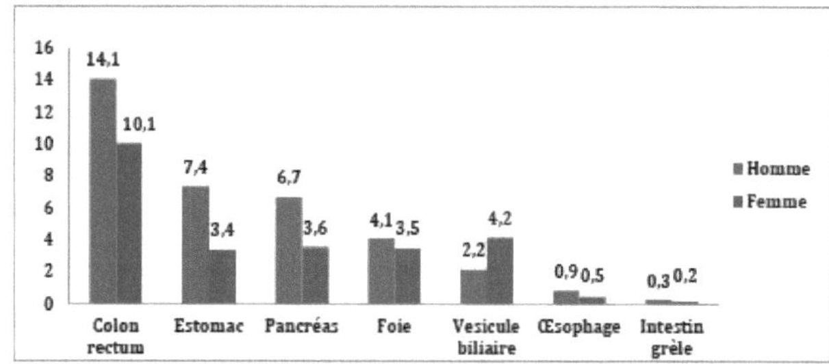

Figure 101. Comparison of mean standardised incidences of different digestive cancers by sex in Souk-Ahras 2016 - 2018.

In Souk-Ahras, in men, CRC, stomach cancer and especially pancreatic cancer have high incidences, whereas in women, VB cancer comes after CRC.

3.5.14. Wilaya of El Oued 2016 - 2018 :

3.5.14.1. Proportion of digestive cancers in both sexes, El Oued 2015 - 2018 :

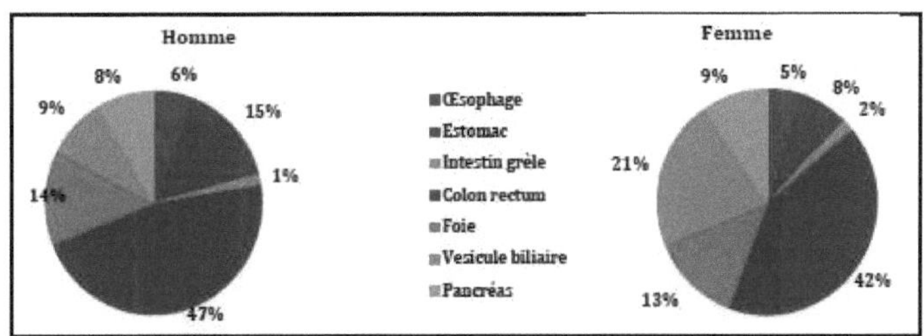

Figure 102. Distribution of digestive cancers in both sexes, El Oued 2015 - 2018.

emeIn this wilaya, in women, VB cancer ranks second after CRC with 21%.

Liver cancer represents, in both sexes, significant proportions (14% in men and 13% in women) which allows liver cancer to be ranked in the 3rd positioneme .

1.1.1.2. . Incidence of all digestive cancers in both sexes, El Oued 2015-2018 :

Table 48: Crude, standardised incidence and rank of all digestive cancers in El Oued, 2015 - 2018 in both sexes.

Year	2015		2016		2017		2018	
Gender	H	F	H	F	H	F	H	F
Number of cases	50	58	88	66	65	57	84	70
Gross rate	12,3	14,8	20,9	16,4	15,3	16,1	18,9	16,4
Rate Standardise*	/	/	37,9	29,4	29,2	28,2	35,9	29,1
% / other cancers	22,3	21,8	24,9	18,9	27,0	24,8	29,8	24,1

538 new cases of digestive cancer were registered between 2015 and 2018 with a slight male predominance. The crude and standardised incidences are 18.9 and 16.4 for men and 35.9 and 29.1 for women respectively in 2018.

1.1.1.3. . Standardised incidence of digestive cancers by location in El Oued, 2015 - 2018

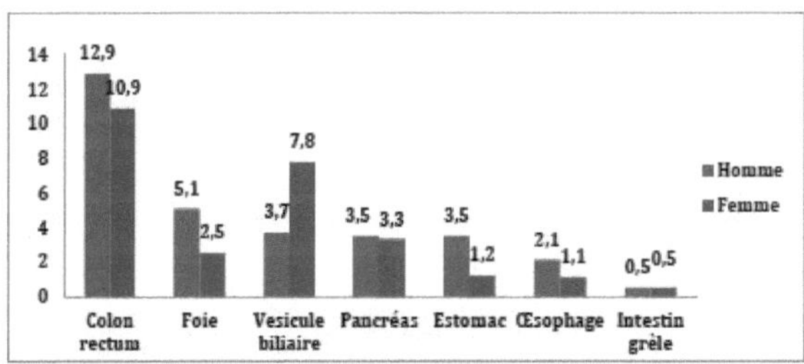

Figure 103. Comparison of mean standardised incidences of different digestive cancers by sex in El Oued 2015 - 2018.

According to the data of the register of this wilaya, in women, the incidence of VB cancer and liver cancer is important.

3.5.15. Wilaya of Tebessa 2016 - 2018

3.5.15.1. 1. Proportion of digestive cancers in both sexes, Tebessa 2016 - 2018 :

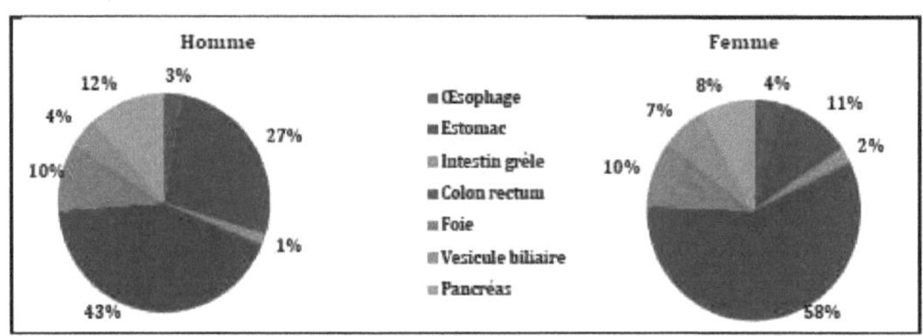

Figure 104. Distribution of digestive cancers in both sexes, Tebessa 2016 - 2018.

CRC ranks first for both sexes with 43% in men and 58% in women, followed by gastric cancer (27% in men and 11% in women).

emeIn men, pancreatic cancer is in 3rd place with 12%, while liver cancer is in the same position in women with 10%. Cancer of the resophagus and the small intestine are less frequent.

3.5.15.2. Incidence of all digestive cancers in both sexes, Tebessa 2016-2018:

Table 49: Crude, standardised incidence and rank of all digestive cancers in Tebessa, 2016 - 2018 in both sexes.

Year	2016		2017		2018	
Gender	H	F	H	F	H	F
Number of cases	32	29	61	54	45	52
Gross rate	8,4	7,7	16,1	14,5	11,7	13,7
Rate Standardise*	11,6	11,5	23,3	21,9	16,2	19,9
% / other cancers	26,1	15,6	26,3	15,6	24,5	17,3

273 cases of digestive cancers were recorded between 2016 and 2018, affecting both men and women. The crude and standardised incidences are respectively

In 2017, the figures were 16.1 and 23.3 for men and 14.5 and 21.9 for women, but they are decreasing in 2018.
Digestive cancers represent 25% of male cancers and 15% of female cancers.

3.5.15.3. Standardised incidence of digestive cancers by location in Tebessa, 2016 - 2018

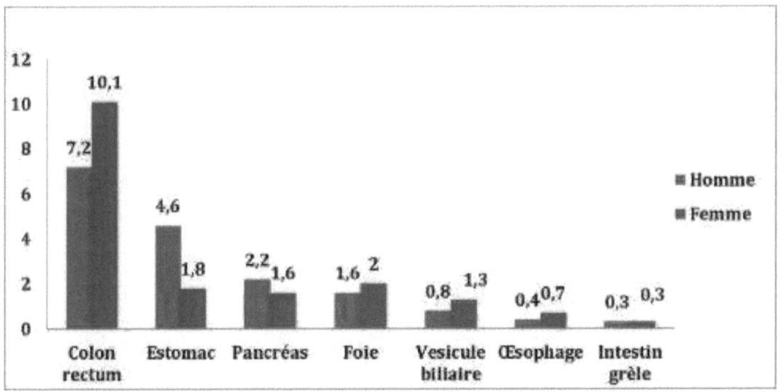

Figure 105. Comparison of mean standardised incidences of different digestive cancers by sex in Tebessa 2016 - 2018.

According to the data of the register of this wilaya, the incidence of the various digestive cancers is moderately low, the highest being CRC.

3.5.16. Wilaya of Mila 2015 - 2018

Incidence of all digestive cancers in both sexes, Mila 2015-2018

Table 50: Crude and standardised incidence and rank of all digestive cancers in Mila, 2015 - 2018 for both sexes.

Year	2015		2016		2017		2018	
Gender	H	F	H	F	H	F	H	F
Number of cases	28	22	32	30	102	83	30	49
Gross rate	6,4	5,1	7,3	6,9	22,7	18,7	6,5	10,8
Rate Standardise*	8,8	6,7	9,1	9,1	42,8	32,7	9,4	14,0
% / other cancers	25	11,7	30,9	13,2	36,2	17,9	36,0	29,1

3.5.17. Wilaya of Khenchela 2015 -2018

Incidence of all digestive cancers in both sexes, Khenchela 2015-2018:

Table 51: Crude and standardised incidence and rank of all digestive cancers in Khenchela, 2015 - 2018 in both sexes.

Year	2015		2016		2017		2018	
Gender	H	F	H	F	H	F	H	F
Number of cases	38	38	14	14	15	10	4	9
Gross rate	16,8	17,4	6,0	6,1	6,0	4,3	1,6	3,8
Rate Standardise*	22,5	25,0	7,4	9,1	10,4	7,4	2,3	7,3
% / other cancers	34,2	25	48,1	20,6	22,7	7,9	10,5	8,8

3.5.18. Wilaya of Guelma 2016 -2018

Incidence of all digestive cancers in both sexes, Guelma 2016 2018:

Table 52: Crude, standardised and ranked incidence of all digestive cancers in Guelma, 2016 - 2018 in both sexes.

Year	2016		2017		2018	
Gender	H	F	H	F	H	F
Number of cases	42	38	31	25	54	62
Gross rate	15,1	13,8	11,0	8,9	19,4	22,7
Rate Standardise*	16	15,3	11,1	8,4	23,5	26,4
% / other cancers	29,1	28,3	34,8	23,6	23,2	26,4

3.5.19. Wilaya of M'sila 2017 -2018

Incidence of all digestive cancers in both sexes, M'sila 2017 2018:

Table 53: Crude, standardised and rank incidences of all digestive cancers in M'sila, 2017 - 2018 in both sexes.

Year	2017		2018	
Gender	H	F	H	F
Number of cases	103	76	49	41
Gross rate	15,9	10,8	7,1	6,4
Rate Standardise*	25,0	19,1	11,1	9,9
% / other cancers	32	10,8	40,6	22,8

Given the constraints identified in the registers of the last four wilayas: Mila, Khenchela, Guelma and M'sila. The impacts are either quite low or vary sharply in an illogical way and do not reflect the reality at all.

3.6. Impact projections

3.6.1. Projections of the incidence of all digestive cancers in the eastern and south-eastern region of Algeria

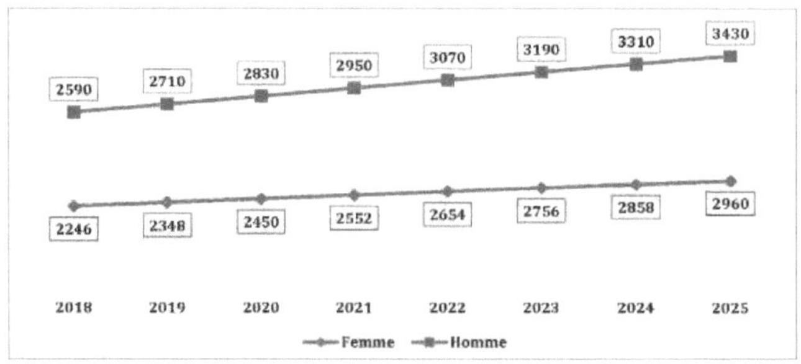

Figure 106. Projections of the number of new cases of digestive cancers for both sexes, ESEA region 2018 - 2025.

For all digestive cancer sites, the number of cases in this region will increase from 4836 new cases in 2018 to 6390 new cases in 2025.

This increase concerns both sexes, but is more marked in men, where the number of new cases will rise from 2590 in 2018 to 3430 in 2025.

3.6.2. Projections of the incidence of all digestive cancers in some wilayas of the East and South-East region of Algeria

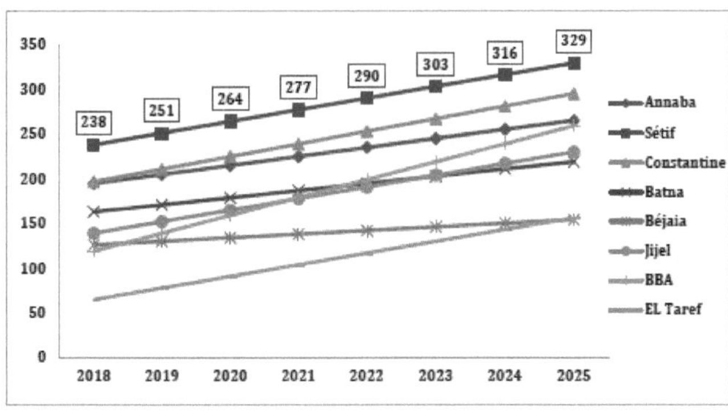

Projections of the number of new cases of digestive cancers from some registries in the ESEA region in men 2018 - 2025.

It should be noted that the number of new cases of all digestive cancers in men will rapidly increase in the wilaya of Setif, Constantine, Jijel, El Taref and especially BBA. Contrary to the other wilayas where the number of new cases will remain stable or almost stable, notably in Bejaia.

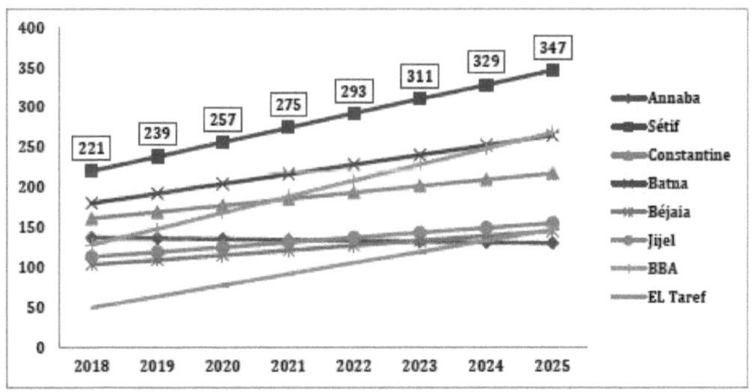

Figure 107. Projections of the number of new cases of digestive cancers from some ESEA registries in women 2018 - 2025.

It should be noted that the number of new cases of all digestive cancers in women will increase rapidly in the wilayas of Setif, Batna, El Taref and especially BBA. Contrary to the other wilayas where the number of new cases will remain stable or almost in Bejaia, or will decrease in Annaba.

3.6.3. Projections of the incidence of the main digestive cancers in the eastern and south-eastern region of Algeria

3.6.3.1. Projections of CRC incidence in the East and South-East region of Algeria

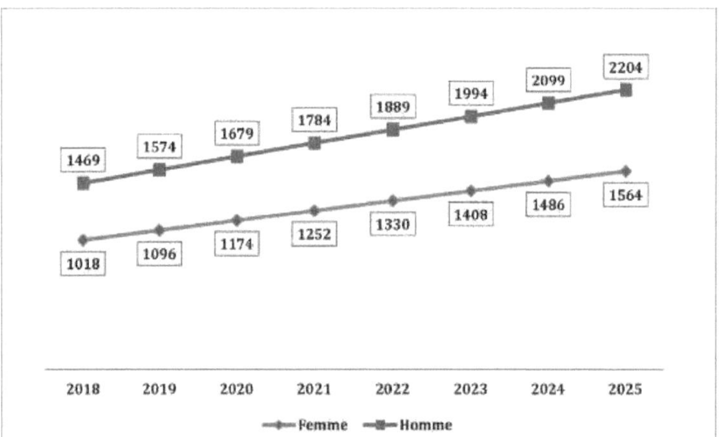

Figure 109. Projections of new CRC cases for both sexes, ESEA Region 2018 - 2025.

The number of CRC cases in this region will increase from 2487 new cases in 2018 to 3768 new cases in 2025.

This increase affects both sexes but is more pronounced in men, with the number of new cases rising from 1469 in 2018 to 2204 in 2025.

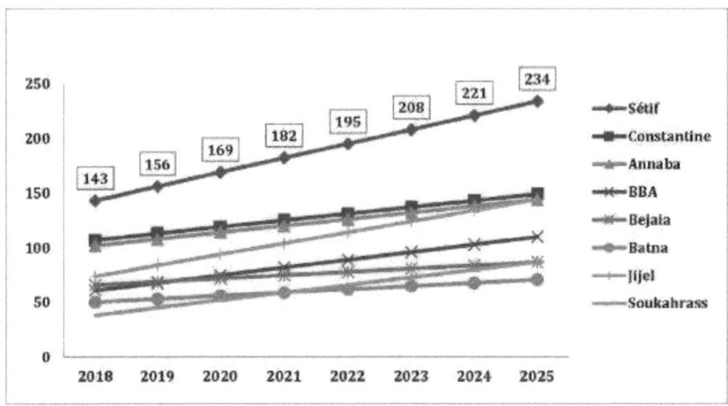

Figure 110. Projections of the number of new CRC cases in selected wilayas of the ESEA network in men 2018 - 2025.

In men, the number of new CRC cases will increase very rapidly in the wilaya of Setif, from 143 in 2018 to 234 in 2025, in Jijel and Souk-Ahras also but with a limited number of cases.
In the other wilayas the number of new cases will gradually increase.

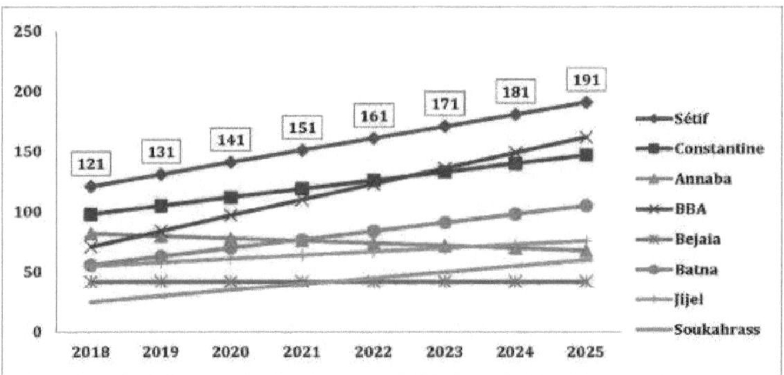

Figure 111. Projections of the number of new CRC cases in selected wilayas of the ESEA region in women 2018 - 2025.

In women, the number of new CRC cases will increase rapidly in the wilaya of Setif from 121 in 2018 to 191 in 2025, in Jijel and Souk-Ahras also but with a limited number of cases.

In the other wilayas, the number of new cases will increase progressively except for Annaba and Bejaia where it will remain stable or it may decrease.

3.6.3.2. Projections of the incidence of stomach cancer in the eastern and south-eastern region of Algeria

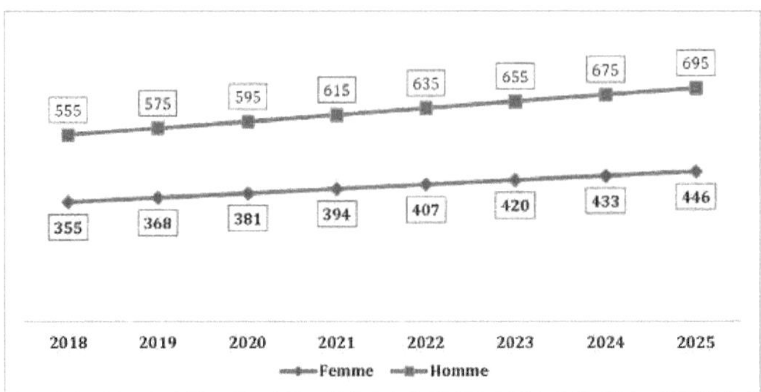

Figure 112. Projected number of new cases of stomach cancer by sex, ESAE region 2018 - 2025

The number of stomach cancer cases in this region will increase from 901 new cases in 2018 to 1141 new cases in 2025.

This gradual increase concerns both sexes but is more significant in men, with the number of new cases rising from 555 in 2018 to 695 in 2025.

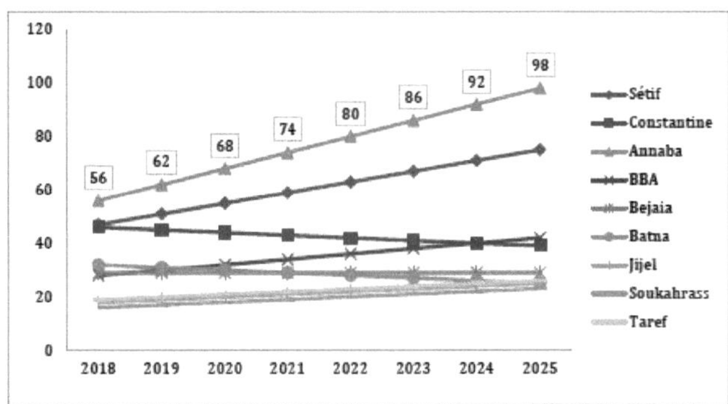

Figure 113. Projections of the number of new cases of stomach cancer in selected wilayas of the ESEA network in men 2018 - 2025.

In men, the number of new cases of gastric cancer will increase in Setif, and in the wilaya of Annaba where it will rise from 56 in 2018 to 98 in 2025.

In the wilayas of Souk-Ahras, Jijel, BBA and EL Taref, the number of new cases will increase progressively at a rate of less than 1%.but in Constantine and Batna and Bejaia, the number will decrease.

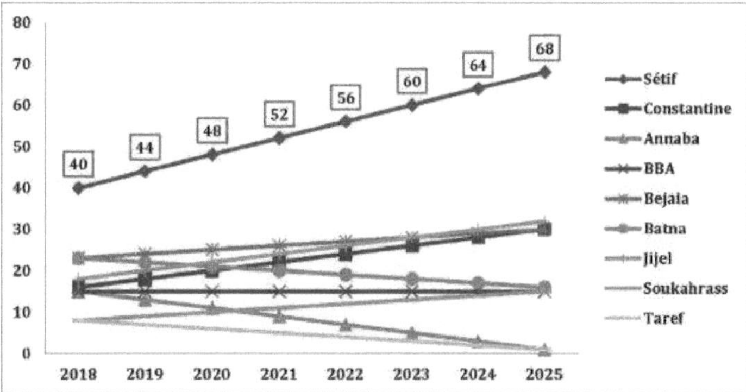

Figure 11. Projections of the number of new cases of stomach cancer in women in selected wilayas of the ESEA network 2018 - 2025.

We note that the number of new cases of stomach cancer in women will increase rapidly in the wilaya of Setif, from 40 in 2018 to 68 in 2025. In Annaba, El Taref and Batna the number will decrease. For the other wilayas, the number of new cases will remain almost stable or will slightly increase.

4. DISCUSSION

At the end of this exhaustive study on the epidemiology of digestive cancers in the East and South-East Algerian region, covering 19 wilayas of the country, i.e. a population of 16 826 987 inhabitants. A number of points and questions deserve to be raised and discussed. The aim of this regional study was to determine the epidemiological coverage of cancer registration and to provide incidence data for the different digestive cancer sites on the one hand, and to define the evolutionary trend and geographical distribution of these cancers in the East and South-East region of the country, during the period 2014 to 2018 on the other.

4.1. Cancer registration coverage

Before 2014, there were only 8 registers nationwide, of which 3 were valid, those of Setif in the east, Algiers in the centre and Oran in the west of the country.

Since 2014, and after the implementation of the strategic axis N°6 of the cancer plan 2015 -2019 in accordance with the ministerial decree N°22 of 18 February 2014, regarding the institutionalization of population registries, the generalization of cancer registration in all wilayas of the country and the establishment of a national cancer network[10] , The rate of registration coverage of the East and South East Network from valid registers has continued to grow until it reached 90% in 2017, covering more than one third of the Algerian population, i.e. 15,528,870 inhabitants. This rate reflects the good functioning and coordination of the various registers in this region, despite the difficulties encountered.

Table 54. Comparison of registration coverage with other countries :

Country	Coverage rate
ESEA Network	**90%**
National registers	
Tunisia	60 %
Egypt	31%
Libya	21%
Morocco	20%
Register networks	
Francim de France (14 registers)	24 %
Airtum from Italy	40 %
United Kingdom	55 %
(CDC, SEER) of the United States (JRC) from Canada and (BKRG) from Germany	Between 70 and 90

Source: Incidence data from the National Cancer Registry Network, Algeria, 2015; Revue El hakim

The coverage rate of the East and South-East region is the highest in Africa, of the Maghreb and Middle East countries (Tunisia 60%, Egypt 31%, Libya 21%, Morocco 20%)[176] . The coverage rate of neighbouring countries remains quite low despite the initiation of national cancer control plans.

Tunisia is the first country in the Maghreb to join the WHO's cancer control strategy. Since 2006, Tunisia has committed to successive five-year anti-cancer plans. The first one covered the period 2006-2010, the second one the period 2010-2015 and the last one the years 2015-2019[177] . Despite the implementation of these three plans, the coverage rate remains low, and this is linked to various shortcomings, the main ones being

- The existence of only 3 registers;
- lack of comprehensiveness and research around registers, harmonisation of publications;
- The data management software is also different (the Canreg5 software is only used by the Sousse Cancer Registry);
- Difficulties in accessing data from certain sources, particularly in the private sector.

In 2010, Morocco joined the international strategy for cancer control and mobilized for the elaboration and implementation of a National Cancer Prevention and Control Plan (NCCP) for the period 2010-2019, thanks to the partnership between the Lalla Salma Association for Cancer Control (ALSC) and WHO for the promotion of cancer prevention and care[178] .

The coverage of cancer registration in the East and South-East region of Algeria, compared to European networks, is higher than the *Francim* network of France with 14 registers (24%), the *Airtum* network of Italy (40%) and the United Kingdom (55%). This coverage is comparable to that of other developed countries' networks: (CDC, SEER) of the United States, (CCR) of Canada and (BKRG) of Germany which are between 70 and 90%, and to other national registries such as Ireland, Austria, Denmark, Croatia, and Finland (80 - 100%)[179, 180, 181] .

4.2. Overall incidence data :

Cancer is a burden borne by the world, with net variations in the incidence of the disease[179] . Cancer in Algeria is now a priority public health concern.

The number of new cases registered in the South-East region for all sites in both sexes in 2017 was 19033, with a standardised rate in relation to the world population of around 178 per 100,000 inhabitants, these incidence rates tend to exceed the ceiling of the data in North Africa which are close to the data collected in the so-called "medium incidence" countries as defined by the International Agency for Research on Cancer (the standardised incidence rate is between 100 and 150 new cases per 100.000 people at risk), these incidences tend to be close to the incidences recorded in Southern Europe. They remain, however, far below those recorded in Western and Northern European and North American countries, which exceed 300 new cases per 100,000 people (USA: 352.2, UK: 319.2, Italy: 290.6, France: 344.1). They are moving away from countries with a low HDI (115 per 100,000 inhabitants)[13] .

Table 55: Annual crude incidence rates by sex -Algeria: 2015-2017

Male incidence rate* Female incidence rate Average incidence rate

2015	100,	2111,8	106,0
2016	104,	1132,7	118,4
2017	93,7131,7		112,2

Source: Epidemiological Surveillance of Cancer: National Preliminary Results, AJSH

The incidence of female cancers is higher with a standardised rate of 195.4 per 100 000 inhabitants, with a small variability in the different registers of the network. Similarly for Morocco where the predominance is female, in Tunisia cancer is more frequent in men than in women[176, 181] .

Worldwide, cancer is predominantly male with a standardised rate of 218.6 for men and 182.6 per 100,000 for women, in France the sex ratio is 1.2[13, 20] .

Table 56: The five most frequent cancers in terms of incidence in the Maghreb

	Gender	1st	2nd	3rd	4th	5th
Tunisia	**H**	Lung	Bladder	JRC	Prostate	NHL*.
	F	Breast	JRC	Cervix uteri	NHL	Lymphoma
Algeria	**H**	JRC	Lung	Prostate	Bladder	Stomach
	F	Breast	JRC	Thyroid	Cervix uteri	Ovary
Morocco	**H**	Lung	Prostate	JRC	Bladder	NHL
	F	Breast	Cervix uteri	JRC	Thyroid	NHL
Region	**H**	Lung	JRC	Prostate	Bladder	Stomach
ESEA	**F**	Breast	JRC	Thyroid	Cervix uteri	Stomach

Source: Globocan 2018

* Non-Hodgkin's lymphoma

The most frequent cancers in the same region, in terms of incidence, in men are lung, colorectal, prostate and bladder cancers. In women, breast cancer dominates, accounting for 42.4%, followed by colorectal, thyroid and cervical cancers.

In Morocco, in men, prostate cancer comes in 2eme . The same position for women is for cervical cancer.

In Tunisia, bladder cancer ranks 2eme in men.

These cancers are often diagnosed at a late stage and the trend in incidence is increasing in the three Maghreb countries[176] .

Worldwide, lung cancer is the most common cancer in men, accounting for 15.5% of all newly diagnosed cases in 2018. The top three cancers (lung, prostate and colorectal) account for 44.4% of all cancers. Other common cancers such as stomach and liver cancer account for more than 5%.

Breast cancer was the most common cancer in women worldwide, accounting for 25.4% of all newly diagnosed cases in 2018.

The three main cancers (breast, colorectal and lung) account for 43.9% of all cancers.

Cervical cancer is the fourth most common cancer in women, accounting for 6.9% of all newly diagnosed cases in 2018.

4.3. Incidence data for all digestive cancers

Colorectal cancers are the most common digestive cancers in both sexes, followed by stomach and bowel cancers in women and pancreatic cancer in men. Cancers of the liver, resophagus and small intestine are less frequent in this region in both sexes.

emeHowever, globally, liver cancer ranks third after CRC and stomach cancer for all sexes ***(Globocan* 2018)**.

The number of cases, crude incidence and standardised incidence of digestive cancers in the East and South-East region are increasing at a rate of about 5% per year, mainly due to the increase in the incidence of CRC, which accounts for a large proportion of these cancers. From 2014 to 2018, the incidence rose from 26.1 to 40.2 per 100,000 men and from 22.1 to 34.1 per 100,000 women. The East and South-East region is in the so-called medium risk regions for digestive cancer.

Digestive cancers are predominant in men, accounting for almost one third of all cancers in men and 18.8% in women.

The specific incidence rates of all digestive cancers increase progressively with age from the age of 40 onwards in both sexes, and are rare in young subjects.

4.5. Incidence data by location

4.5.1. Colorectal cancer

emeIn our study region, CRC is the third most common cancer after breast and lung cancer, the second most common cancer site (16% in men and 11.2% in women) and the most common digestive site (about 50% of these cancers) in both sexes.
In men, these cancers are clearly on the increase, from a crude incidence rate of 9.6 and a standardised incidence rate of 13.5 per 100,000 inhabitants in 2014 to a crude incidence rate of 16.8 and a standardised incidence rate of 21.9 per 100,000 inhabitants in 2018 (MVA = 10%). In women, there has also been a marked increase in both crude and standardised incidence rates.

Table 57. Comparison of CRC incidence in the East and South East region with other countries for both sexes:
According to the NCCRN, colorectal cancer affects both men and women. It became the leading male cancer in 2017, surpassing lung cancer, which had been the leading male cancer since the beginning of cancer registration in Algeria (15,2) (182).

Country	**Male**	**Woman**
Denmark	45,9	36,6
Spain	45,2	23,3
France	36,9	24,8
USA	28,8	22,6
Region ESEA	**19,3**	**18,2**
South Africa	18,1	12,0
Algeria	16,4	13,4
Saudi Arabia	16,1	10,9
Iran	14,6	11,1
Tunisia	14,0	11,7
Kuwait	13,1	11,9
Morocco	12,9	9,9
Egypt	6,6	6,3
India	5,8	3,1

Source :Globocan 2018

The standardised incidence of CRC in the East and South-East region is high compared to that observed in the Maghreb countries (Tunisia, Morocco), Egypt and other Arab countries[176] . But it is still lower than in developed countries considered as high risk regions for CRC such as the USA, Canada, Australia[183] and in Europe (in France, the standardised incidence rates are 34.0 cases per 100,000 population).

The ratio of cases per 100,000 person-years in men to cases per 100,000 person-years in women is 23.9 (male/female ratio 1.4). These geographical differences are thought to be due to differences in environment and dietary habits, which are imposed against a background of genetically determined susceptibility [20]

Colon and rectal cancers share the same risk factors. The responsibility of lifestyle and environment in the development of colorectal cancer is proven. The protective effect of a high-fibre diet and the detrimental effect of overweight/obesity, sedentary lifestyle, smoking, alcohol and high consumption of processed meat are well established. Effective engagement and mobilisation of policy makers and stakeholders is essential. Genetic factors are probably intertwined with environmental factors. The risk is also increased in people with a history of adenoma or colorectal cancer and in cases of extensive inflammatory colitis. This risk is very high in people with a hereditary gene mutation: Lynch syndrome and familial adenomatous polyposis. Hence the importance of mass screening for CRC in this region to limit its progression.

In the East and South East region, CRC affects men 1.1 times more than women (worldwide CRC affects men more than women with a sex ratio of 1.47), this excess risk is probably related to the difference in exposure to risk factors such as lifestyle, diet, smoking, obesity and exposure to restrogens[14] .

The risk of colon and rectal cancer increases with age, and over the age of 45 it is considered sufficiently high for this cancer to be the subject of an organised screening programme. The median age at diagnosis in 2017 is 63 years for men and 62 years for women, which is lower than in European countries, e.g. in France the median age at diagnosis in 2018 is 71 years for men and 73 years for women, however, a recent increase in CRC incidence is observed in young adults in the USA, Canada, Australia and parts of Asia[20, 144] .

4.5.2. Stomach cancer :

Stomach cancer remains the third most common cause of cancer deaths worldwide[13] . emeemeAccording to data recorded in the East and South-East region over the five years, stomach cancer is the 5th most diagnosed cancer, ranking 2nd after CRC in both sexes.

Stomach cancer accounts for 6% of male cancers and 3% of female cancers.

Table 58. Comparison of the incidence of gastric cancer in the East and South-East region with other countries for both sexes:

In both sexes, the incidence rate is stable with periods of slight non-significant increases, the mean crude and standardised rates were 5.9 and 8.2 per 100,000 for men and 3.9 and 5.1 per 100,000 for women respectively.

Country	Male	Woman
Iran	22,4	12,5
Spain	9,2	4,3
Region ESEA	**8,2**	**5,1**
Morocco	8,0	3,7
France	7,2	2,9
Algeria	6,9	4,4
India	6,2	2,9
Denmark	6,0	2,5
USA	5,6	2,8
South Africa	4,9	2,5
Tunisia	4,1	2,4
Egypt	3,1	2,7
Saudi Arabia	3,0	2,2
Kuwait	2,9	2,4

This incidence is higher than that estimated by the NCCSR (7.4 in men) and is close to that of Morocco. Compared to developed countries, it is higher than in the USA, Denmark and France, where the incidence is 6.3 in men and 2.7 in women[20] . This difference is mainly related to the control of the main risk factors in developed countries, which are *Helicobacter pylori* infection, smoking and diet[20] .

In the East and South East region, gastric cancer is more common in men than in women, affecting 1.6 times more men than women. Worldwide, gastric cancer is 2.2 times more likely to be diagnosed in men than in women. In France, the sex ratio is 2.3[20] . One possible explanation is that the protective effect of restrogen may reduce the risk of gastric cancer in women[96] . Other causes, such as differences in diet and occupational exposure, may contribute to the increased incidence of gastric cancer in men[97] . The risk of gastric cancer is reduced by delayed menopause and increased fertility. An increased risk may be observed with anti-restrogen drugs, for example tamoxifen[184] . Post-menopausal incidence of gastric cancer in women shows a similar pattern to that in men, but with a 10-15 year delay[97] .

The risk of stomach cancer increases with age from the age of 40 onwards, the median age at diagnosis in the region is 67 for men and 62 for women, which is lower than the estimated age in France of 71 for men and 75 for women. In the USA, stomach cancer occurs most often in people over the age of 55. Most people diagnosed with stomach cancer are between 60 and 70 years old[95] .

4.5.3. Gallbladder and HGV cancer

Gallbladder cancer is an uncommon cancer, with an estimated incidence of 2.1 in men and 2.4 in women per 100,000 person-years in 2018. High incidence areas are in South America and Asia[13] . Europe is a medium-risk area, with an incidence of 3.0 and 2.6 per 100,000 in men and women respectively[14] , with Eastern European countries, particularly the Czech Republic and Slovakia, having the highest incidence rates.

In the East and South East region, VB and VBEH cancer ranks 3[eme] among digestive cancers in women and 4[eme] in men. In 2018, the standardised incidence is increasing in both sexes, it was 4.9 in women and 2.8 in men with a sex ratio of 0.55. The incidence compared with that of European countries is higher than in France, where it is 2.1 in men (up by 1.1%) and 1.4 in women (down by 1.2%). This fact leads to a reversal of the sex ratio over time, which has risen from 0.8 to 1.5[20] . The gender gap tends to be higher in endemic areas and lower in low incidence areas. At the European level, rates remain stable in both men and women[185]. Several studies have shown sometimes divergent results regarding the evolution of the incidence[20].

According to the results for the region, the median age at diagnosis is 67 years for men and 62 years for women. There is a strong increase in incidence rates from the age of 45 for both sexes but it is more marked in women.

The main common risk factors for these cancers are lithiasis, especially for gallbladder cancer, obesity and diabetes[186]. The role of smoking, alcohol or hormonal and reproductive history in women has also been mentioned.

4.5.4. Pancreatic cancer

[eme]Pancreatic cancer accounts for 9.8% of all digestive cancers and is the third most common digestive cancer in men and the fourth most common in women. Its average incidence during the study period in this region was 4.0 per 100,000 population in men and 2.8 per 100,000 population in women with a slight male predominance. The incidence is higher than the national incidence or that of neighbouring countries estimated by ***Globocan*** in 2018, as well as for other African countries where the incidence does not exceed 2 per 100,000 population. However, the incidence is still very low compared to that in developed countries where pancreatic cancer is a public health problem, being the 7[eme] cause of cancer deaths (fourth in the USA). Data regularly published by the *International Association of Cancer of Cancer Registries* (IACR) do not show significant disparities in the incidence of pancreatic cancer in Europe[187].

Table 59. Comparison of the incidence of pancreatic cancer in the East and South East region with other countries for both sexes:

Country	**Male**	**Woman**
France	10,8	7,1
USA	9,0	6,6
Denmark	8,5	7,0
Spain	7,9	5,4
Region ESEA	**5,0**	**3,2**
South Africa	5,0	3,6
Egypt	4,8	2,6
Iran	4,7	2,9
Tunisia	4,5	2,5
Kuwait	4,1	4,3
Morocco	3,9	2,5
Algeria	2,9	1,8
Saudi Arabia	2,6	1,6
India	0,81	0,88

Source :Globocan 2018

In France, it is the third most common cancer in men and the second most common cancer in women among digestive cancers. The standardised incidence rates are 11.0 in men and 7.7 in women with a sex ratio of 1.4[20].

The reason for these differences in the incidence of this cancer between countries is not entirely clear. However, it is possible that the environment and/or exposure to certain risk factors explain the observed geographical variation in pancreatic cancer incidence. For example, some results indicate that smoking may have an effect on these differences[188]. On the other hand, other studies explain them by dietary style and obesity[189]. It should be noted that diagnostic tools and the change in use of various diagnostic modalities vary between developed and

undeveloped geographical areas[190] . In addition, some differences in incidence can be attributed to the quality of registries, including coverage, completeness and accuracy, which vary from country to country[191] . The reasons for the higher incidence of pancreatic cancer in men are still not well understood. Women are less exposed to the environmental risk factors that are responsible for the development of this cancer. Women are less prone to this type of malignancy[192] .
Apart from the small proportion of pancreatic cancer occurring in the context of familial genetic predisposition (5-10% of cases), smoking and obesity are the most established environmental risk factors. Excessive consumption of alcohol, red meat, increased abdominal fat, and occupational exposures to X-rays and ygenium occupational exposures to X- and y-rays and Thorium-232 are strongly suspected to play a role in the occurrence of pancreatic cancer (*World Cancer Research Fund / American Institute for Cancer Research (WCRF / AICR)* classification). Part of the increase could be attributed to the increasing prevalence of obesity in populations. Epidemiological studies are needed to better explain these trends.

The incidence rate in the East and South East region for both sexes increases with age. Pancreatic cancer is rarely diagnosed before the age of 55 and can be defined as a disease of older populations as the highest incidence is reported in people over 70 years of age, with similar variations in different countries[39] .

4.5.5. Liver cancer

Liver cancer represents only 5% of digestive cancers, it is the fifth most common cancer in men and women. The male/female ratio is 1.26 (the male predominance is not really confirmed).
Table 60. Comparison of liver cancer incidence in the East and South East region with other countries for both sexes:

Country	Male		Woman
Egypt	33,8		22,7
France	12,4	3,3	
USA	10,4	3,7	
Spain	10,4	2,5	
Iran	7,5	6,1	
South Africa	6,9	3,1	
Denmark	6,8	3,1	
Saudi Arabia	6,8	3,3	
Kuwait	5,4	4,1	
Tunisia	4,7	4,0	
Morocco	3,9	2,8	
India	3,6	1,6	
Region ESEA	**2,2**	**1,9**	
Algeria	1,7	1,6	

Source :Globocan 2018

In the East and South-East region, the incidence of primary liver cancer (the data available to us do not allow us to distinguish between hepatocellular carcinoma, which is the most frequent histological type, and intra-hepatic cholangiocarcinoma) reaches 2.6 per 100,000 inhabitants for both sexes, and is very different from that of North African countries such as Morocco, Tunisia and above all Egypt, where the incidence is 33.8 for men and 22.7 for women.) It is also far from

In developed countries, where the incidence of liver cancer is high, it is more marked in men than in women. Sub-Saharan Africa and East Asia account for more than 80% of HCC worldwide, with 20 cases per 100,000 people, Southern Europe (10 to 20 cases per 100,000 people), America (North and South), Northern Europe and Oceania (less than 5 cases per 100,000 people).

This geographical variation in the distribution of incidences is mainly related to the level of endemicity of viral hepatitis B and C, to the increase in incidence of chronic liver diseases related to alcohol, metabolic steatopathies[193] , and to the improved management of cirrhosis[194] .

The median age at diagnosis in 2017 was 63 for men and 72 for women. These cancers are rare before the age of 55 in both sexes.

4.5.6. Resophageal and small bowel cancer

These cancers are rarely diagnosed in this region, representing less than 3% of digestive cancers.

Table 61. Comparison of the incidence of resophageal cancer in the East and South-East region with other countries for both sexes:

Country	Male	Woman
South Africa	9,5	4,9
France	6,1	1,5
India	6,1	3,4
Denmark	6,0	2,1
USA	4,8	1,1
Iran	4,6	3,5
Spain	4,0	0,7
Egypt	2,1	1,7
Kuwait	1,5	0,93
Morocco	1,4	0,98
Region ESEA	**1,1**	**0,7**
Saudi Arabia	1,1	0,91
Tunisia	0,75	0,64
Algeria	0,6	0,52

Source :Globocan 2018

The national or regional incidence of resophageal cancer (the available data do not allow us to distinguish between squamous cell carcinoma, which is the most frequent histological type, and adenocarcinoma) was low compared to the various Western, Arab and even neighbouring countries. It was around 1.1 per 100 000 population for men and 0.7 per 100 000 population for women. South Africa has a very high rate for both sexes, exceeding even that of developed countries. The main risk factors for this cancer are alcohol consumption and smoking for squamous cell carcinoma, obesity and gastroesophageal reflux disease for adenocarcinoma[195,196] .

In 2018, the East and South East region recorded crude and standardised rates of graft bowel cancer of 0.7 and 0.8 per 100,000 population for men and 0.6 and 0.8 per 100,000 population for women. The rates reported, compared with those of European countries, are slightly lower than those of France, which is 1.6 cases per 100,000 people for men and 1.0 cases per 100,000 people for women, and Denmark, which is 1.4 per 100,000 people.

The main known risk factors are hereditary predisposing conditions including familial adenomatous polyposis, Lynch syndrome, and inflammatory bowel diseases such as Crohn's disease and celiac disease[147,197] . Because of the rarity of this cancer, relative knowledge is limited and epidemiological studies are difficult.

4.6. Geographical variations

The incidence data from each registry and the cartographic aspect make it possible to compare the incidence of digestive cancers between the wilayas covered by a cancer registry and to search for possible disparities in geographical distribution.
CRC ranks first for all wilayas in the region. The incidence rates of colorectal cancer were higher in Annaba and Jijel (> 20 per 100 000 inhabitants), for both sexes, than in the rest of the region, and these rates tend to be close to the incidences recorded in Europe[20] .

In men, during the study period, high CRC incidence rates were observed in El Taref which is a wilaya very close to Annaba, Setif, Bejaia and Constantine (between 17 and 20). For the other northern wilayas, the variations in incidence are not very marked.
Among women, the wilayas of BBA and Setif have high rates of CRC (about 20).
Gastric cancer came in 2eme position in most of the wilayas, with a very high incidence in Annaba, El Taref and BBA which record very high incidence rates especially in men (> 9), they exceed those observed in the rest of the region, they even exceed those of the European countries and North America
In women, only EL Taref and BBA have high rates of stomach cancer and it is low compared to men (< 5 per 100 000 women for most wilayas).
Incidence rates of CRC and stomach cancer are very significantly different between the north and south of the network. These differences are far too large to be attributed to a recruitment bias in the south, which is related to inaccessibility to care and the absence of cancer centres, and can be attributed to the level of exposure and possible risk factors that may cause these cancers. If these differences were confirmed and if they were found in the other networks, they would constitute an important characteristic of the epidemiological profile of these two digestive localisations in Algeria.
The rank of gastric cancer is different in only a few wilayas, where we find other digestive localisations which occupy the second position, it is the case of the wilaya of El Oued in the South-East which registers a high incidence of gall bladder cancer and VBEH in women associated with an exceptional increase in hepatic cancer (> a 5 in men), with a high probability of intra- and extrahepatic cholangiocarinoma which share the same risk factors, namely lithiasis.) The wilaya of Souk-Ahras also recorded high rates of pancreatic cancer (> 6.5), liver cancer and VB.
The incidence of biliary tract cancer is highest in El Oued, Batna and Jijel (>7 per 100,000 women), exceeding the global figures.
Cancers of the resophagus and the small intestine have a low incidence in almost all the wilayas of the eastern and south-eastern region of Algeria.
This analysis shows significant variability and requires epidemiological studies, particularly on risk factors.

4.7. Trends in digestive cancers :

From 2018 to 2025, the number of new cases of digestive cancers will increase by 32%, or 6390 new cases in the ESEA region, this increase is observed in most registries but with a variable speed, it is more important in Jijel, Setif, Constantine, El Taref, Batna and BBA. The downward trend in some registers may be related to registration problems or to a recruitment bias.

The rapid progression of these cancers and its concomitance with the important social changes experienced in Algeria during the last two decades have contributed to the increase in exposure to proven risk factors for this cancer. Among the most important risk factors are: the important change in the type of diet in connection with a massive rural exodus, a change in lifestyle leading to reduced individual mobility and a profound modification of the environment with rapid and polluting industrialisation.

The number of CRC cases in this region will increase from 2487 new cases in 2018 to 3768 new cases in 2025. This increase concerns both sexes but is more pronounced in men, the number of new cases will rise from 1469 in 2018 to 2204 in 2025 and concerns most wilayas but especially Setif where the number of cases will reach 420 in 2025.

The incidence of CRC will continue to rise in this region if no preventive measures are taken; one measure is to reduce the prevalence of the main risk factors, namely smoking and obesity, the other is early detection of precancerous lesions. This is in contrast to developed countries where there has been a decline in CRC incidence. A decrease was first observed in the United States since the 1970s, followed by a decline in the incidence of colon cancer since the mid-1980s. This decrease in incidence will appear later in France in the mid-1990s and 2000s respectively for rectal and colon cancer in men, while the incidence has remained stable in women (20)

The introduction of organised screening and resection of precancerous lesions partly explains this decrease. A decrease in the prevalence of exposure to certain environmental factors (such as smoking) could also explain these favourable trends in these countries.

The number of stomach cancer cases in this region will increase slightly (less than 25%), reaching 1141 new cases in 2025. This gradual increase concerns both sexes but is more marked in men. There is a disparity between the different wilayas and both sexes.

In men, stomach cancer will increase in the wilayas of Annaba and Setif. In the wilayas of Souk-Ahras, Jijel, BBA and EL Taref, the number of new cases will gradually increase, but will decrease in Constantine, Batna and Bejaia.

In women, the number of new cases of stomach cancer will increase rapidly in the wilaya of Setif. On the other hand it will decrease in Annaba, El Taref and Batna.

In the other wilayas, for both sexes, the number of new cases will remain almost stable or will increase slightly.

Worldwide, the incidence of stomach cancer has steadily decreased over the past 50 years. These declines have preceded the successful reduction of *Helicobacter pylori* infection and are probably attributable to changes in food preservation, such as pickling of vegetables, smoking and meat processing. The decline has also been caused by the increased availability of fresh fruit and vegetables(198) .

The second major factor in the decline of gastric cancer is the success of prevention and treatment of *Helicobacter pylori* infections in most developing countries(198) , up to 90% of non-cardia gastric cancer cases are attributable to this germ.

In France, its incidence is constantly decreasing. The decrease in the incidence of stomach cancer is attributed to the decrease in the prevalence of *Helicobacter pylori,* linked to better hygiene, access to drinking water, the use of antibiotics, and a decrease in tobacco consumption(20) .

Table 62. Projections of the incidence of the 2 main digestive cancers in Algeria: 2015-2025

	Gross rates 2015	New cases 2015	New cases 2020	New cases 2025
Male				
JRC	10,3	2034	2668	3710
Stomach	4,7	928	899	888
Woman				
JRC	12,2	2410	3128	4141
Stomach	3,4	731	878	1075

Source: Epidemiological Surveillance of Cancer: National Preliminary Results, AJSH

5. Constraints and biases of the study

Our study critically evaluated this cancer surveillance system by identifying and analysing both quantitative and qualitative limitations and weaknesses. Despite the wide coverage and quality of the data, four registries were excluded from the incidence estimates of disgestive cancers in the region. Several methodological limitations were identified:

Difficulties in accessing the database of the different registries for further study (depending on histological type, degree of differentiation and grade of cancer, data sources ....).

Due to the limitations of the standardisation method, the standardised incidence rates are calculated in relation to a global reference population. However, the structure of the world population is older than that of the Algerian population. Furthermore, the standardised rates will tend to reflect more the rates observed in the older age groups than those observed in the younger age groups.

The absence of the exact address of the patients, especially for data from laboratories or private anatomopathology practices, thus leading to a recruitment bias. This explains, for example, why the wilaya of Annaba has a very high incidence rate for practically all digestive cancers, unlike the neighbouring wilayas, particularly Skikda, where the incidence is low. This can be explained by the competence and excellent services in Annaba in the area of diagnosis and treatment of cancers.

These shortcomings (lack of information) do not allow a study to be carried out on the distribution of cases according to the communes of each wilaya and to compare the incidence of digestive cancers between urban and rural areas.

For the estimation of the incidence of the region, the populations (2014-2018) of the different registers have been estimated from ONS data. The latter are based on growth rates from the last Algerian population census (2008) (between 2.09 and 2.16).

The population data for the incidences from the registers are not precise for the majority of cases, which may explain the random fluctuations in incidence rates by wilaya and by year.

For the 2018 notifications, there was a decrease in the registration of cases, which is believed to be linked to the outbreak of the Covid 19 pandemic (given that all medical staff were mobilised to deal with the pandemic), which led to a delay in the transmission of information and in the estimation of the regional incidence of digestive cancers.

The specific difficulties of registers :

- Structural problems for the wilayas of Bejaia and M'sila.
- Human resources problems and instability of the register team in M'sila, OEB, Constantine, Batna, Khenchela, Skikda and El Taref.

This study allowed us to determine the incidence, age distribution and geographical variations of the different digestive cancer sites. This epidemiological profile reflects the situation in our country, but it would be necessary to compare it with those of other networks (centre, west).

6. PROSPECTS AND RECOMMENDATIONS

The synthesis of all the available data on the incidence of digestive cancers in the East and South-East region converges towards the evidence that these cancers have become a public health priority in our country. These data will also allow us to propose recommendations for a strategy of control in terms of primary prevention, screening and early diagnosis and management.

> To propose strategies for the fight against digestive cancers

Primary prevention of digestive cancers, particularly in terms of reducing the prevalence and level of risk factors, remains the main strategy for controlling these cancers. Public awareness is essential to ensure health promotion and the adoption of a healthy lifestyle and the fight against risk factors such as tobacco use, poor diet, sedentariness and obesity. Effective engagement and mobilisation of policy makers and stakeholders is essential.

1. Reduce tobacco consumption.

The main interventions are :

- Increase taxes against tobacco.
- Strengthen the reduction of access to tobacco products.
- Designating tobacco as a dangerous product: warning on cigarette packs.
- Ban the promotion of all tobacco products: advertising, attractive packaging, mass display of products at the point of sale, etc.

2. Improving physical activity and nutrition

- Promoting the production of health-promoting foods.
- To develop and implement a physical education programme for schools where such a programme is officially lacking (preschool, primary and university)
- To promote basic healthy eating and health education among parents of preschool and school children.
- Reviewing the core curricula for nutrition and health education for teachers in schools and colleges
- Promote the consumption of fruit and vegetables. Mediterranean-style diet, rich in fibre and low in red meat and fat.
- Revise the physical education and sports curriculum (time and activities) in secondary education.
- Strengthen or integrate physical activity in public spaces.
- To strengthen the provision and equipment of sports facilities in schools, universities, professional and public areas.

2. **For biliary and hepatic cancers,** which are frequent in Oued and Souk-Ahras, it is necessary to reinforce primary prevention measures, i.e. early diagnosis and management of lithiasis and vaccination against hepatitis B.

3. The search for and subsequent eradication of *Helicobacter pylori* is recognised as an effective method of prevention against the development of stomach cancer.

4. Reducing environmental exposure to cancer-causing substances

- To raise awareness and improve the knowledge of health professionals about cancer-environment risk and means of prevention.

• Improving the assessment, monitoring and control of cancer-causing environmental substances.

5. Develop and disseminate public health messages to raise awareness of evidence-based environmental cancer risks and inform people of specific measures to reduce or eliminate exposures.

The urgency of organised screening in the most affected wilayas, especially for colorectal cancer (Annaba, Jijel, BBA, Setif, Constantine, El Taref and Souk-Ahras), given its high frequency and seriousness, and the fact that it is preceded in 80% of cases by an adenomatous polyp, which can prevent its malignant transformation. A controlled population-based study by Faivre et al in 2004 showed a reduction in colorectal cancer mortality of almost 16% after 11 years of follow-up. Other studies show that the reduction in colorectal cancer mortality after 10 and 7 years of screening respectively was 18% in Denmark and 14% in England.

For gastric cancer, as its frequency is still high in some wilayas (Annaba for both sexes, El Taref, BBA, Batna, Setif, Constantine and Souk-Ahras for men), endoscopic exploration is recommended for subjects at risk.

For pancreatic cancer, given its seriousness and high frequency, especially in Souk-Ahras and Batna (an ASR that is close to Western countries), targeted screening for precancerous lesions is necessary (intraepithelial neoplasia, TIPMP) **(see Chapter 3).**

Given the importance of the familial form of some digestive cancers, it is necessary to :

- To promote target screening.
- To create oncogenetic consultations that would take care of these families according to a well-defined algorithm and in conformity with the recommendations of the learned societies.
- Include trained dieticians in these consultations to specifically advise these high and very high risk individuals on dietary risk factors and primary prevention.
- Long-term investment in oncogenetic research projects, to establish a genetic profile of our population.

By 2025, the number of new cases of digestive cancers will increase by 32%, or 6390 new cases in the ESEA region. It will be necessary to anticipate and prepare for the reception and improvement of the care of cancer patients, by -The creation of new specialised centres

-The regular organisation of continuing medical education days on digestive cancers (from diagnosis to management) for general practitioners.

These days should be led by the different specialists: gastroenterologists, internists, surgeons, oncologists, radiotherapists, anatomopathologists, epidemiologists, psychologists and nutritionists.

> **Evaluation of the performance of the existing plan and identification of research priorities.**

In fact, the implementation of the activities of the cancer plan in its various components must be accompanied by monitoring and evaluation of the effectiveness of the actions undertaken in order to identify the needs for intervention and to assess the impact of the measures taken to combat cancer. In the absence of such data, it would be difficult to define priorities, to assess the effectiveness of preventive measures and of the health care system, to generalise good practice, to detect inequalities and to trace the effects of risk factors.

Evaluate, critique and reinvigorate the multisectoral programme to address risk factors for non-communicable diseases. Their effectiveness should not be judged solely on the impact of the programme on reductions in the prevalence of the target risk factors.

> **For better epidemiological surveillance :**

- Establish a hospital information system. and set up hospital cancer registries which aim to meet not only the needs of hospital administration and hospital cancer programmes, but above all the needs of the patients themselves.

- The development and improvement of population-based registries for surveillance, planning and research in cancer control strategy must remain a priority.
- Accurate and regularly published population data is a necessity in the organisation of a population register.
- Multiplication of data sources, i.e. private clinics, radiology centres (especially for liver cancer), laboratories and health insurance funds.
- Strengthen the registry teams with human resources and secure and sustain the funding of the registry.
- Improving the surveillance system for causes of death.
- Consolidation of registers not yet valid (training, updating of registration tools, supervision, evaluation)
- Promotion and valorisation of cancer registries (Visibility and Publications IARC5, WHO)
- Database of reliable data on cancer epidemiology (Planning for public health and scientific research development)
- Trend and projection studies would be of great value for cancer control planning and strategy.
- Survival studies would be reliable indicators of the effectiveness of patient management and therefore of the efficiency of the health system. The Setif and Annaba registries have participated in the international survival studies CONCORD 1, 2 and 3. The efficient registries of the network should participate in the next CONCORD studies.

Analytical epidemiological studies on the risk factors of the main locations:
Scientific research in cancer has become a priority, justified by the seriousness of the disease and the increasing trend for certain locations. Mapping allows the detection of areas of high incidence for each cancer and consequently to prioritise them for research and funding of health programmes. While research on protective factors towards low incidence areas.
The north-south gradient provides a model for etiological research in CRC and gastric cancer. It is desirable to start with prevalence surveys on key risk and protective factors, ecological surveys followed by case-control studies and meta-analyses.

CONCLUSION

Despite the shortcomings, the creation of the national network of cancer registries has enabled Algeria to have, for the first time, sufficient annual data to provide a national incidence of cancers by sex, age group and location.
This initiative constitutes an important advance in the knowledge of these pathologies. The incidence rates of cancers in Algeria and their evolution show that cancer pathology has accompanied the demographic and economic changes experienced by our country over the last two decades. The profound changes in the epidemiological profile of the diseases are largely the consequence of these changes.
The main characteristics of these mutations are

- An improvement in the standard of living of the population with the emergence of a large and increasingly educated middle class;
- A rapid increase in average life expectancy to 75 years in 2017;
- An ageing population with an increase in the proportion of people over 60 in the age pyramid;
- An increase in the proportion of urban dwellers, who now constitute more than 50% of the

general population;

- Major changes in environment, lifestyle and diet;

Given the frequency and severity of digestive cancers, epidemiologists must take a special interest in these cancers. In this context, epidemiological studies are a means to mitigate the magnitude of this worrying situation. Descriptive epidemiological data allow us to know the frequency of the disease, variations over time and to identify risk groups. These data are also useful for making etiological hypotheses, for designing and analysing surveys aimed at identifying the causes of cancers, and for defining and evaluating prevention programmes.

The present study is a first comprehensive study on the epidemiology of digestive cancers in the East and South East region of the country, covering 19 wilayas. This represents about half of the Algerian population, over a period of 5 years, from 2014 to 2018.
Cancer registration coverage has reached 90% of the population in the East and Southeast regions. It is comparable to that of countries with well functioning population registries.

These results on the incidence of digestive cancers observed in the different wilayas deserve to be analysed, in order to answer various questions and to put forward hypotheses on the increase in the incidence of these cancers, especially that of colorectal cancer. The incidence data, their evolution and their local and regional specificities will make it possible to put forward hypotheses and research avenues for analytical epidemiological studies on the risk factors. These data and their follow-up will be the basis for epidemiological surveillance of cancer in Algeria.

In addition, trend and projection studies will be of great value for cancer control planning and strategy. Also, survival studies will be reliable indicators of the effectiveness of patient care and thus of the efficiency of the health system.
The development and improvement of population-based registries for surveillance, planning and research in cancer control strategy should remain a priority.

All indicators show that the continuous increase in the incidence of digestive cancers, especially CRC, is unstoppable. The later they are diagnosed, the higher the human and financial costs.

Given the multiple Western influences of diet on digestive cancers, the aim should also be to encourage the consumption of locally grown vegetables, fruit and produce and to avoid Western eating habits, and return to the Mediterranean diet.
Early detection of cancer through early diagnosis and population screening should be a priority to reduce the high incidence of late-stage digestive cancers, and thus increase survival rates, which remain very low compared to Western countries.
The measures of the 2015-2019 Cancer Plan must be converted into actions adapted to the field and must be evaluated.
In the fight against cancer, the role of cancer associations is becoming important in reducing the incidence of the disease and mortality. The synergy between the strategies of the public authorities and the effective daily actions of the associations has become essential for an effective fight against cancer. The dynamic, day-to-day commitment of associations has an important impact on prevention and the quality of life of patients. Associations do not have the right to remain passive in the face of this epidemiological transition.

REFERENCES

1. Cancer Plan 2015 - 2019 first edition .ANDS. National Cancer Plan 2015-2019, new strategic vision focused on the disease, October2014. http://www.sante.gov.dz/plan cancer/plan_national_cancer.pdf

2. Working group of the international association of cancer registries. Guidelines on confidentiality for population-based cancer registration. IARC internal report No.2004/03. 2004.

3. Ferlay J, Soerjomataram I, Ervik M, Dikshit R, Eser S, Mathers C et al. GLOBOCAN 2012 v1.0, Cancer Incidence and Mortality Worldwide: IARC Cancer Base No. 11 Lyon, France: International Agency for Research on Cancer; 2013.

4. Fact Sheet No. 297. March 2017, Geneva, WHO 2017.

5. GBD 2015 Risk Factors Collaborators. Global, regional, and national comparative risk assessment of 79 behavioural, environmental and occupational, and metabolic risks or clusters of risks, 1990-2015: a systematic analysis for the Global Burden of Disease Study 2015. Lancet. 2016 Oct; 388 (10053):1659-1724.

6. Berrino F., Capocaccia R., Esteve J., Gatta G., Hakulinen T., Micheli A., Sant M.and Verdecchia A., 1999. Survival of cancer patients in Europe: The Eurocare 2 study. IARC. Sci. Pub. No. 151, Lyon.

7. Laszlo Herszenyi, Zsolt Tulassay Epidemiology of gastrointestinal and liver tumors .European Review for Medical and Pharmacological Sciences 2010; 14: 249258.

8. IARC (Intenatinal Agency for Research on Cancer) 2015.

9. Bouvier AM, Remontet L, Jougla E et al Incidence of gastrointestinal cancers in France. Gastroenterol Clin Biol 2004; 28:877-881.

10. Ministerial order on the creation, functioning and organisation of the population cancer register. Available at Portal.org/sites/default/files/resources/arret%C3%A9%20registre%20cancer%2020 14.pdf

11. Arrete No 98 du 27Septembre 2015 fixant le Reseau national des registres de cancer. Ministere de la Sante et de la reforme Hospitaliere.

12. Global burden of 5 major types of gastrointestinal cancer Melina Arnold , Christian C. Abnet, Rachel E. Neale, Edward L. Giovannucci, Katherine A. McGlynn, Freddie Bray.

13. Bray F, Ferlay J, Soerjomataram I, et al. Global cancer statistics 2018: GLOBOCAN estimates of global incidence and mortality for 36 cancers in 185 countries. CA Cancer J Clin. 2018; 68: 394-424.

14. Ferlay J, Ervik M, Lam F, et al. World Cancer Observatory: Cancer Today. Lyon, France: International Agency for Research on Cancer; Available at: https://gco.iarc.fr/today , accessed 2 November 2018.

15. Global Burden of Disease Cancer Collaboration, Fitzmaurice C, Allen C, et al. Global, regional, and national cancer incidence, mortality, years of life lost, years lived with disability, and disability-adjusted life years for 32 cancer groups, 1990 to 2015: a systematic analysis for the study of the global burden of disease. JAMA Oncol 2017; 3: 524.

16. Ward EM, Sherman RL, Henley SJ, et al. Annual report to the Nation on the state of cancer, featuring cancer in men and women aged 20 to 49 years. J Natl Cancer Inst 2019; 111: 1279.

17. Siegel RL, Miller KD, Jemal A. Cancer statistics, 2020. CA Cancer J Clin 2020; 70: 7.

18. Jemal A, Bray F, Centre MM, et al. Global cancer statistics. CA Cancer J Clin 2011; 61:69.

19. Centre MM, Jemal A, Ward E. International trends in colorectal cancer incidence rates. Biomarkers of Cancer Epidemiol Prec. 2009; 18: 1688.

20. National estimates of cancer incidence and mortality in metropolitan France between 1990 and 2018 volume 1: solid tumours / colon and rectum)

21. Niger Med J. 2017 May-June; 58 (3): 87-91.doi: 10.4103 / 0300-1652.234076 Emergence of colorectal cancer in West Africa: accepting the inevitable David O. Irabor

22. Centre MM, Jemal A, Smith RA, Ward E. Global variations in colorectal cancer. CA Cancer J

Clin 2009; 59: 366.
23. Siegel RL, Miller KD, Jemal A. Colorectal cancer mortality rates among adults aged 20 to 54 years in the United States, 1970-2014. JAMA 2017; 318: 572.
24. Third atlas of the cancer register of Setif 1986-2016.
25. Hamdi cherif M, Bouharati K,Kara L, Hamouda D, Fouatih Z. cancers in algeria epidemiological data from the national network of cancer registries,2015. World Cancer Day, Setif, Feb 2017.
26. Balakrishnan M, George R, Sharma A, Graham DY. Changing trends in stomach cancer throughout the world. Curr Gastroenterol Rep. 2017;19:36.
27. Digestive Cancer Aid and Research booklet stomach 2016.
28. Howlader NA, Krapcho M, Miller D, et al. SEER Cancer Statistics Review, 19752014. Bethesda, MD: National Cancer Institute cancer; https://seer.cancer.gov/csr/1975_2014/ , based on the SEER data submission of November 2016, published on the SEER website, April 2017.
29. Cancer Research UK https://www.cancer research uk.org/health- professional/cancer-statistics/statistics-by-cancer-type/stomach- cancer/survival#heading-Two . October 2018.
30. Gatto M, Bragazzi MC, Semeraro R, Napoli C, Gentile R, Torrice A, et al. Cholangiocarcinoma: update and future perspectives. Dig Liver Dis. 2010 Apr;42(4):253-260.
31. Blechacz BR, Gores GJ. Cholangiocarcinoma. Clin Liver Dis. 2008 Feb; 12 (1): 13150. ix.
32. Patel T. Cholangiocarcinoma. Nat Clin Pract Gastroenterol Hepatol. 2006 Jan; 3 (1): 33-42.
33. Shaib Y, El-Serag HB. The epidemiology of cholangiocarcinoma. Semin Liver Dis. 2004 May;24(2):115-125.
34. Khan SA, Toledano MB, SD Taylor-Robinson. Epidemiology, risk factors and pathogenesis of cholangiocarcinoma. HPB (Oxford) 2008; 10 (2): 77-82.
35. Torre LA, Siegel RL, Islami F, et al. Global burden and trends in mortality from gallbladder and other biliary cancers. Clin Gastroenterol Hepatol. 2018; 16: 427-437.
36. GLOBOCAN 2012. Estimated cancer incidence mortality and prevalence worldwide in 2012. International Agency for Research on Cancer. World HealthOrganization,http://globocan.iarc.fr/
37. Raimondi S. Epidemiology of pancreatic cancer: An overview. Nat Rev Gastroenterol Hepatol 2009;6:699708
38. Swiss Cancer League. (2012).pancreatic cancer in 2014: epidemiology and screening Swiss Medical Journal.
39. Ferlay J EM, Lam F, Colombet M, Mery L, Pineros M, Znaor A, Soerjomataram I, World Cancer Observatory: cancer today. Lyon, France: International Agency for Research on Cancer; Available at: https://gco.iarc.fr/today , accessed 5 October 2018.
40. SEER cancer statistics review, 1975-2013 [Internet]. National Cancer Institute, Bethesda, MD. 2016. Available at: https://seer.cancer.gov/csr/1975 2015/ . Accessed on 5 October 2018.
41. Jessica L Petrick, Andrea A Florio, Ariana Znaor, David Ruggieri, Mathieu Laversanne, Christian S Alvarez, Jacques Ferlay, Patricia C Valery, Freddie Bray, Katherine A McGlynnInternational trends in hepatocellular carcinoma incidence, 1978-2012 PMID: 31597196.PMCID: PMC7470451.
42. Katherine A. McGlynn, Jessica L. Petrick, and Hashem B. El-Serag. Epidemiology of Hepatocellular Carcinoma. REVIEWS HEPATOLOGY, VOL. 73, NO. S1, 2021
43. Petrick JL, Florio AA, Znaor A, Ruggieri D, Laversanne M, Alvarez CS, et al. International trends in hepatocellular carcinoma incidence, 1978-2012. Int J Cancer 2019 Oct 9. https://doi.org/10.1002/ijc.32723.
44. Statistics adapted from the American Cancer Society (ACS) publication, Cancer Facts & Figures 2021, and the ACS website (sources accessed January 2021).
45. Blot W, McLaughlin J, Fraumeni J. Esophageal cancer. In Cancer epidemiology and

prevention, Schottenfeld D, Fraumeni J. Oxford: Oxford University Press, 2006:697-706 **46.** Pennathur A, Gibson MK, Jobe BA, Luketich JD. Resophageal carcinoma. Lancet. 2013; 381: 400-412.
47. Zhang Y. Epidemiology of resophageal cancer. World J. Gastroenterol. 2013; 19 : 5598-5606.
48. Zhang HZ, Jin GF, Shen HB. Epidemiological differences in resophageal cancer between Asian and Western populations. Chin J Cancer. 2012; 31: 281-286.
49. Wheeler JB, Reed CE. Epidemiology of resophageal cancer. Surg Clin North Am. 2012; 92: 1077-1087.
50. Bojesen RD, Riis LB, Hogdall E, Nielsen OH, Jess T. Inflammatory Bowel Disease and Small Bowel Cancer Risk,Clinical Characteristics, and Histopathology: A Population-Based Study. Clin Gastroenterol Hepatol. Dec 2017; 15(12):1900-1907.e2.
51. Kurniawan N, Ruther C, Steinbruck I, Baltes P, Hagenmuller F, Keuchel M. Tumours in the Small Bowel. Video Journal and Encyclopedia of GI Endoscopy. Jan 2014;1(3-4):632-5.
52. Reynolds I, Healy P, Mcnamara DA. Malignant tumours of the small intestine. Surgeon. Oct 2014;12(5):263-70.
53. Lepage C, Bouvier A-M, Manfredi S, Dancourt V, Faivre J. Incidence and management of primary malignant small bowel cancers: a well-defined French population study. Am JGastroenterol. Dec 2006;101(12):2826-32.
54. Curado MP, Edwards B, Shin HR, Storm H, Ferlay J, Heanue M, Boyle P. Cancer Incidence in Five Continents Vol. IX. Lyon: IARC, IARC Scientific Publication, No. 160; 2007.
55. Haselkorn T, Whittemore AS, Lilienfeld DE. Incidence of graft bowel cancer in the United States and worldwide: geographic, temporal, and racial differences. Cancer Takes Control. 2005; 16: 781-787.
56. Weiderpass E, Pukkala E. Temporal trends in socio-economic differences in incidence rates of gastrointestinal tract cancers in Finland. BMC Gastroenterol. 2006; 6 : 41.
57. Schottenfeld D, Beebe-Dimmer JL, Vigneau FD. Epidemiology and pathogenesis of neoplasia in the gut. Ann Epidemiol. 2009; 19: 58-69.
58. Bilimoria KY, DJ Bentrem, Wayne JD, Ko CY, Bennett CL, Talamonti MS. Transplanted bowel cancer in the United States: changes in epidemiology, treatment, and survival over the past 20 years. Ann Surg. 2009; 249 : 63-71.
59. Shack LG, Wood HE, Kang JY, Brewster DH, Quinn MJ, Maxwell JD, Majeed A. Graft bowel cancer in England, Wales and Scotland: temporal trends in incidence, mortality and survival. Aliment Pharmacol Ther. 2006; 23 : 1297-1306.
60. Screening and prevention of colorectal cancer Update of the referential of practices and of the periodic health examination (PSE) June 2013 (HAS) INVS and INCa.
61. Cancer of the colon and rectum. Brochure produced in collaboration with Dr Guy Launoy, Pr Helene Sancho-Garnier and Dr Franfoise May-Levin, Dr Jean-Claude Arnal, Updated February 2008: Dr Henri Bastien. Research Information - prevention - screening. Actions for patients and their relatives (la ligue contre le cancer) page 34.
62. Cirt N, d'halluin Pierre Nicolas, Branger B, Corbinais S, Thirouard AS, Floch L, Poirier JY, Bretagne Jean-Franfois, Heresbach Denis. **Societe savante** des maladies et cancers de l'appareil digestif (SNFGE).
63. Andrew.R, Donnai.D Genetique medicale : de la biologie a la pratique clinique ; page : 323 France : Groupe de Boeck ; 2008
64. ARC Foundation for Cancer Research. On the Fondation ARC website:www.fondation-arc.org Edition: August 2014 brochure cancer CCR **65.** www.les données.e-cancer.fr, fiche indicateur 98.
66. Potter JD, Slattery ML, Bostick RM, Gapstur SM. Colon cancer: a review of the epidemiology. Epidemiology 1993; 15(2):499-545.
67. Bueno de Mesquita HB, Jansen J, Taal BG. Dikke darm- en endeldarmkanker.

In:Rijksinstituut voor Volksgezondheid en Milieuhygiëne, editor. Volksgezondheid toekomst verkenning. De gezondheidstoestand van de Nederlandse bevolking in de periode 1950-2010. Bilthoven: Rijksinstituut voor Volksgezondheid en Milieuhygiëne, 1993: 265-272.
68. Ransohoff DF, Lang CA. Screening for colorectal cancer. New England Journal of Medicine 1991; 325:37-41.
69. Levin B. Colorectal Cancer Screening. Cancer 1993; 72:1056-1060.
70. BUECHER.B, DE PAUW.A Les formes hereditaires des cancers colorectaux La Rev de Med Intern, septembre 2012; 33 (9) :471-474
71. Bonaiti-Pellie.C, Eisinger.F, Feingold.J, Frebourg.T, Grandjouan.S, Lasset.C, Laurent-Puig.P, Lecuru.F, Millat.B, Sobol.H, Gilles.T, Olschwang.S Hereditary predisposition to colorectal cancer Gastroenterol Clin Biol, 2005; 29: 701-710
72. SAURIN.J-CPolyposis other than familial adenomatous polyposis Assangaise de Formation Medicale Continue en Hepato-Gastro-enterologie: Paris; 2008 **73.** WCRF/AICR (2017). Continuous Update Project Report. Diet, nutrition, physical activity and colorectal cancer. Washington (DC), USA: American Institute for Cancer Research. Available from: https://wcrf.org/ colorectal-cancer-2017.
74. IARC handbooks of cancer prevention. Colorectal cancer screening. Volume 17.
75. Harris R. Global epidemiology of cancer. Burlington, MA: Jones Bartlett; 2016.
76. Aune D, Chan DS, Lau R, Vieira R, Greenwood DC, Kampman E, et al (2011). Dietary fibre, whole grains, and risk of colorectal cancer: systematic review and doseresponse meta-analysis of prospective studies. BMJ, 343:d6617. doi:10.1136/bmj.d6617 PMID:22074852
77. Norat T, Scoccianti C, Boutron-Ruault M-C, Anderson A, Berrino F, Cecchini M, et al.(2015). European Code Against Cancer 4th Edition: diet and cancer Cancer Epidemiol, 39(Suppl 1):S56-66. doi:10.1016/j. canep.2014.12.016 PMID:26164653.
78. Lauby-Secretan B, Scoccianti C, Loomis D, Grosse Y, Bianchini F, Straif K; International Agency for Research on Cancer Handbook Working Group (2016). Body fatness and cancer - viewpoint of the IARC Working Group. N Engl J Med, 375(8):794-8.doi:10.1056/NEJMsr1606602 PMID:27557308.
79. Anderson AS, Key TJ, Norat T, Scoccianti C, Cecchini M, Berrino F, et al (2015). European Code Against Cancer 4th Edition: obesity, body fatness and cancer. Cancer Epidemiol, 39(Suppl 1):S34-45. doi:10.1016/j.canep.2015.01.017 PMID:26205840.
80. Boyle T, Keegel T, Bull F, Heyworth J, Fritschi L (2012). Physical activity and risks of proximal and distal colon cancers: a systematic review and meta-analysis. J Natl Cancer Inst, 104(20):1548-61. doi:10.1093/jnci/djs354 .PMID:22914790
81. Mahmood S, MacInnis RJ, English DR, Karahalios A, Lynch BM (2017). Domainspecific physical activity and sedentary behaviour in relation to colon and rectal cancer risk: a systematic review and meta-analysis. IntJ Epidemiol, 46(6):1797-813. doi:10.1093/ije/dyx137 PMID:29025130
82. Robsahm TE, Aagnes B, Hjartaker A, Langseth H, Bray FI, Larsen IK (2013). Body mass index, physical activity, and colorectal cancer by anatomical subsites: a systematic review and meta-analysis of cohortstudies. Eur J Cancer Prev, 22(6):492- 505. doi:10.1097/ CEJ.0b013e328360f434 PMID:23591454
83. World Health Organization Bulletin - Cancer and Tobacco
84. Liang PS, Chen TY, Giovannucci E (2009). Cigarette smoking and colorectal cancer incidence and mortality: systematic review and meta-analysis. Int J Cancer, 124(10):2406-15. doi:10.1002/ijc.24191 PMID:19142968.
85. Fedirko V, Tramacere I, Bagnardi V, et al. Alcohol consumption and risk of colorectal cancer: an overall meta-analysis and dose-response of published studies. Ann Oncol 2011; 22: 1958.
86. GiovannucciE. 2004. Alcohol, one-carbon metabolism, and colorectal cancer: recent insights from molecular studies. J Nutr 134: 2475S-81S. INCa 2007

87. Aliyu & Cullen, 2005Evidence for excess colorectal cancer incidence among asbestos-exposed men in the Beta-Carotene and Retinol Efficacy Trial.
88. Fang, 2011.Identification of occupational cancer risks in British Columbia, Canada: a population-based case-control study of 1,155 cases of colon cancer.PMID: 22073015PMCID: PMC3210584.
89. Tsilidis KK, Kasimis JC, Lopez DS et al. Type 2 diabetes and cancer: a general review of meta-analyses of observational studies. BMJ. 2015; 350 : g7607.
90. Jiang Y, Ben Q, Shen H et al. Sugar diabetes and colorectal cancer incidence and mortality: a systematic review and meta-analysis of cohort studies. Eur J Epidemiol. 2011; 26: 863-76.
91. Pang Y, Kartsonaki C, Guo Y et al. Diabetes, plasma glucose, and colorectal cancer incidence in Chinese adults: a prospective study of 0.5 million people. J Epidemiol Commun Health. 2018; 72: 919-25.
92. Nottage K, McFarlane J, Krasin MJ, et al. Secondary colorectal carcinoma after childhood cancer. J Clin Oncol. 2012; 30: 2552-8.
93. Desautels D, Czaykowski P, Nugent Z, et al. Risk of colorectal cancer after prostate cancer diagnosis: a population-based study. Cancer. 2016; 122 : 1254-60.
94. Rawla P, Vellipuram AR, Bandaru SS, Pradeep Raj J. Colon carcinoma presenting as Streptococcus anginosus bacteremia and liver abscess. Gastroenterology Res. 2017; 10: 376-9.
95. Cancer.Net, 01/2019 .ASCO org (american society of clinical oncology).
96. Stomach cancer: a guide for patients - Based on ESMO recommendations - v.2012.2. page 7.
97. Camargo MC, Goto Y, Zabaleta J, et al. Sex hormones, hormonal interventions, and gastric cancer risk: a meta-analysis. Cancer Epidemiol Biomarkers Prev. 2012;21:20- 38.
98. Edgren G, Hjalgrim H, Rostgaard K, et al. Risk of gastric cancer and peptic ulcers in relation to ABO blood type: a cohort study. Am J Epidemiol. 2010;172:1280-5.
99. Surveillance, Epidemiology, and End Results Program Cancer query system: SEER Incidence Statistics (2000-2015) Available at: http://seer.cancer.gov/Accessed October 29, 2018.
100. Derakhshan MH, Malekzadeh R, Watabe H, et al. The combination of gastric atrophy, reflux symptoms and histological subtype indicates two distinct etiologies of gastric cardia cancer. Intestin. 2008; 57: 298-305.
101. Demicco EG, Farris AB, 3eme, Baba Y, et al. The dichotomy in cancerogenesis of the distal resophagus and resophagogastric junction: mucosal-associated adenocarcinoma of the intestinal vs cardiac type. Mod Pathol. 2011; 24: 1177-90.
102. Muriel Genevay, Pierre Hutter, Pierre O. Chappuis, Patrick R. Benusiglio, PierreO. Chappuis Rev Med Suisse 2011; volume 7. 1502-1506.
103. Boland CR, Yurgelun MB. Historical perspective on familial gastric cancer. Cell Mol Gastroenterol Hepatol. 2017; 192-200.
104. Shimoyama T, Fukuda S,Nakasato F, et al. Relation of CagA seropositivity to cagPai phenotype and histological grade of gastritis in patients with Helicobacter Pylori infection. World J Gastroenterol 2005; 11:3751-5.
105. Pakin DM. The global health burden of infection - associated cancers in the year 2002. Int J cancer 2006; 118:3030 - 44.
106. Boysen T, Mohammadi M, Melbye M, et al. EBV-associated gastric carcinoma in high- and low-incidence areas for nasopharyngeal carcinoma. Br J Cancer. 2009;101:530-3.
107. Murphy G, Pfeiffer R, Camargo MC, Rabkin CS. Meta-analysis shows that prevalence of Epstein-Barr virus-positive gastric cancer differs based on sex and anatomic location. Gastroenterology. 2009;137:824-33.
108. World Cancer Research Fund/American Institute for Cancer Research (WCRF/AICR) Continuous Update Project Report: Diet, Nutrition, Physical Activity and Stomach Cancer 2016. Revised 2018. London: World Cancer Research Fund International; 2008.
109. Ladeiras-Lopes R, Pereira AK, Nogueira A, et al. Smoking and gastric cancer: systematic

review and meta-analysis of cohort studies. Cancer Causes Control. 2008;19:689-701.

110. Sadjadi A, Derakhshan MH, Yazdanbod A, et al. Neglected role of hookah and opium in gastric carcinogenesis: a cohort study on risk factors and attributable fractions. Int J Cancer. 2014;134:181-8.

111. Ma K, Baloch Z, He TT, Xia X. Alcohol consumption and gastric cancer risk: a metaanalysis. Med Sci Monit. 2017;23:238-46.

112. Tsugane S, Sasazuki S. Diet and the risk of gastric cancer: review of epidemiological evidence. Gastric Cancer. 2007;10:75-83.

113. Chang CJ, Tu YK, Chen PC, Yang HY. Talc exposure and risk of stomach cancer: systematic review and meta-analysis of occupational cohort studies. J Formos Med Assoc. 2018 doi: 10.1016/j.jfma.2018.07.015.

114. Kamisawa T, Egawa N, Nakajima H, Tsuruta K, Okamoto A, Matsukawa M. Origin of the long common channel based on pancreatographic findings of pancreatomotor dysfunction. Dig Liver Dis. 2005 May; 37 (5): 363-367.

115. Soreide K, Korner H, Havnen J, Soreide JA. Biliary cysts in adults. Br J Surg. 2004 Dec; 91 (12): 1538-1548.

116. Mabrut JY, Bozio G, Hubert C, Gigot JF. Management of congenital biliary cysts. Dig Surg. 2010; 27 (1): 12-18.

117. Kaewpitoon N, Kaewpitoon SJ, Pengsaa P, Sripa B. Opisthorchis viverrini: the cancer-causing human liver fluke. Monde J Gastroenterol. 7 February 2008; 14 (5): 666674.

118. Torbenson M, Yeh MM, Abraham SC. Biliary tract dysplasia in chronic hepatitis C and alcoholic cirrhosis. Suis J Surg Pathol. 2007 Sep; 31 (9): 1410-1413.

119. Zhang BL, He N, Huang YB, Song FJ, Chen KX. ABO blood types and cancer risk: a systematic review and meta-analysis. Asian Pac J Cancer Prev. 2014; 15 (11): 4643-4650. doi: 10.7314 / APJCP.2014.15.11.4643.

120. Duell EJ, Lucenteforte E, Olson SH, Bracci PM, Li D, Risch HA, Silverman DT. et al. Pancreatitis and the risk of pancreatic cancer: a cluster analysis in International Pancreatic Cancer Case-Control Consortium (PanC4) Ann Oncol. 2012; 23 (11): 2964-2970. doi: 10.1093 / annonc / mds140.

121. Ghiorzo P. Genetic predisposition to pancreatic cancer. World J Gastroenterol. 2014; 20 (31): 10778-10789. doi: 10.3748 / wjg.v20.i31.10778.

122. Pelucchi C, Galeone C, Polesel J, Manzari M, Zucchetto A, Talamini R, Franceschi S. et al. Smoking and body mass index and survival in patients with pancreatic cancer. Pancreas. 2014; 43 (1): 47-52. doi: 10. 1097/ MPA.0b013e3182a7c74b.

123. Wang YT, Gou YW, Jin WW, Xiao M, Fang HY. Association between alcohol consumption and pancreatic cancer risk: a dose-response meta-analysis of cohort studies. Cancer BMC. 2016; 16: 212. doi: 10.1186 / s12885-016-2241-1.

124. Rahman F, Cotterchio M, Cleary SP, Gallinger S. Association between alcohol consumption and pancreatic cancer risk: a case-control study. PLoS One. 2015; 10 (4): e0124489. doi: 10.1371 / journal.pone.0124489.

125. Davoodi SH, Malek-Shahabi T, Malekshahi-Moghadam A, Shahbazi R, Esmaeili S. Obesity as an important risk factor for certain types of cancer. Iran J Cancer Prev. 2013; 6 (4): 186-194.

126. Midha S, Chawla S, Garg PK. Modifiable and non-modifiable risk factors for pancreatic cancer: a review. Cancer Lett. 2016; 381 (1): 269-277. doi: 10.1016 / j.canlet.2016.07.022.

127. Huxley R, et al. Type II diabetes and pancreatic cancer: a meta-analysis of 36 studies. British Journal of Cancer. 2005; 92.11 : 2076.

128. Marcin Lener ,Anna Wiechowska-Kozlowska Jozef Kfadny ,Magdalena Muszynska ,Grzegorz Sukiennicki ,Lidia Kubera-Nowakowska &Jan Lubinski. Selenium and the risk of colon, pancreatic and gastric cancersHereditary cancer in clinical practice volume 10, Article number:

A13 (2012)
129. Kew MC. The role of cirrhosis in the etiology of hepatocellular carcinoma. J Gastrointest Cancer. 2014; 45 : 12-21.
130. Toyokuni S. Role of iron in cancerogenesis: cancer as a ferrotoxic disease. Cancer Sci. 2009; 100: 9-16.
131. Olnyk JK, St Pierre TG, Britton RS, Brunt EM, Bacon BR. Duration of hepatic iron exposure increases the risk of significant fibrosis in hereditary hemochromatosis: a new role for magnetic resonance imaging. Suis J Gastroenterol. 2005; 100 : 837-841.
132. Dhamija E, Paul SB, Kedia S. Non-alcoholic fatty liver disease associated with hepatocellular carcinoma: a growing concern . Indian J Med Res. 2019; 149 (1): 9-17. doi: 10.4103 / ijmr.IJMR_1456_17
133. Liver cancer: a guide for patients - Based on ESMO recommendations - v.2014.1page 07.
134. Morgan TR, Mandayam S, Jamal MM. Alcohol and hepatocellular carcinoma. Gastroenterology. 2004; 127 (5 Suppl 1): S87 - S96.
135. Boffetta P, Hashibe M. Alcohol and cancer. Lancet Oncol. 2006; 7: 149-156.
136. Borena W, Strohmaier S, Lukanova A, et al. Metabolic risk factors and primary liver cancer in a prospective study of 578 700 adults. Int J Cancer. 2012; 131 : 193-200.
137. Zhang Y. Epidemiology of resophageal cancer. World J Gastroenterol. 2013; 19 : 5598-5606.
138. Cui R, Kamatani Y, Takahashi A, et al. et al. Functional variants in ADH1B and ALDH2 associated with alcohol and smoking synergistically increase the risk of resophageal cancer. Gastroenterology. 2009 ; 137 :1768- 1775.
139. Hvid-Jensen F, Pedersen L, Drewes AM, SOrensen HT, Funch-Jensen P. Incidence of adenocarcinoma in patients with Barrett's resophagus. N Engl J Med. 2011; **365**:1375-1383.
140. Alcedo J, Ferrandez A, Arenas J, Sopena F, Ortego J, Sainz R, Lanas A. Trends in the diagnosis of Barrett's esophagus in Southern Europe: implications for surveillance. Dis oesophagus. 2009; 22 : 239-248.
141. Resophageal cancer: a guide for patients - Based on ESMO recommendations - v.2012.1 Page 5
142. Mana Jose Domper Arnal , Angel Ferrandez Arenas and Angel Lanas Arbeloa. Resophageal cancer: risk factors, screening and endoscopic treatment in Western and Eastern countries 2015 .PMCID : PMC4499337 PMID : 26185366
143. Renehan AG, Tyson M, Egger M, Heller RF, Zwahlen M. Body mass index and cancer incidence: systematic review and meta-analysis of prospective observational studies. Lancet. 2008; 371: 569-578.
144. Surveillance, Epidemiology and End Results (SEER) Program. SEER * Stat Database: Incidence - SEER 18 Regs Research Data + Hurricane Katrina Impacted Louisiana Cases, Nov 2015 Sub (1973-2013 Varying) -Linked To County Attributes - Total US, 1969-2014 Counties, National Cancer Institute, DCCPS, Surveillance Research Programme, Surveillance Systems Branch, published April 2016, based on November 2015. [(last accessed February 15, 2019)];Available online: https://seer.cancer.gov/statfacts/html/smint.html
145. Shenoy S. Genetic risks and familial associations of small bowel carcinoma. World J. Gastrointest. Oncol. 2016;8:509-519. doi: 10.4251/wjgo.v8.i6.509.
146. Bonadona V., Bonaiti B., Olschwang S., Grandjouan S., Huiart L., Longy M., Guimbaud R., Buecher B., Bignon Y.J., Caron O., et al. Cancer risks associated with germline mutations in MLH1, MSH2, and MSH6 genes in Lynch syndrome. JAMA. 2011;305:2304-2310. doi: 10.1001/jama.2011.743.
147. Bojesen R.D., Riis L.B., Hogdall E., Nielsen O.H., Jess T. Inflammatory Bowel Disease and Small Bowel Cancer Risk, Clinical Characteristics, and Histopathology: A Population-Based Study. Clin. Gastroenterol. Hepatol. 2017;15:1900-1907. doi: 10.1016/j.cgh.2017.06.051.

148. Aparicio T., Manfredi S., Tougeron D., Henriques J., Bouche O., Pezet D., Piessen G., Coriat R., Zaanan A., Legoux J.L., et al. 772PARCAD-NADEGE cohort: Result of a small bowel adenocarcinomas prospective cohort. Ann. Oncol. 2018;29 doi: 10.1093/annonc/mdy282.155.
149. 54. Cross A.J., Leitzmann M.F., Subar A.F., Thompson F.E., Hollenbeck A.R., Schatzkin A. A prospective study of meat and fat intake in relation to small intestinal cancer. Cancer Res. 2008;68:9274-9279. doi: 10.1158/0008-5472.CAN-08-2015.
150. Bagnardi V., Rota M., Botteri E., Tramacere I., Islami F., Fedirko V., Scotti L., Jenab M., Turati F., Pasquali E., et al. Alcohol consumption and site-specific cancer risk: A comprehensive dose-response meta-analysis. Br. J. Cancer. 2015;112:580-593. doi: 10.1038/bjc.2014.579.
151. Boffetta P., Grant E.J., Ozasa K., Tsuji I., Kakizaki M., Nagai M., Nishino Y., You S.L., Yoo K.Y., Yuan J.M., et al. Body mass, tobacco smoking, alcohol drinking and risk of cancer of the small intestine-A pooled analysis of over 500 000 subjects in the Asia Cohort Consortium. Ann. Oncol. 2011;23:1894-1898. doi: 10.1093/annonc/mdr562.
152. Habib R.R., Abdallah S.M., Law M., Kaldor J. Cancer Incidence among Australian Nuclear Industry Workers. J. Occup. Health. 2006;48:358-365. doi: 10.1539/joh.48.358.
153. Fukase K, Kato M, Kikuchi S, Inoue K, Uemura N, Okamoto S, Terao S, Amagai K, Hayashi S, Asaka M, Japan Gast Study Group (2008) Effect of eradication of Helicobacter pylori on incidence of metachronous gastric carcinoma after endoscopic resection of early gastric cancer: an open-label, randomised controlled trial. Lancet372 (9636): 392-397
154. Rothwell PM, Fowkes FG, Belch JF, et al. Effect of daily aspirin on long-term risk of cancer death: analysis of individual patient data from randomised trials. Lancet 2011; 377: 31.
155. Bosetti C, Santucci C, Gallus S, Martinetti M, La Vecchia C. Aspirin and the risk of colorectal and other digestive tract cancers: an updated meta-analysis through 2019. Ann Oncol. 2020 May;31(5):558-568. doi: 10.1016/j.annonc.2020.02.012. Epub 2020 Apr 1. PMID: 32272209.
156. Samadder NJ, Neklason DW, Boucher KM, et al. Effect Of Sulindac And Erlotinib vs Placebo On Duodenal Neoplasia In Familial Adenomatous Polyposis: A Randomized Clinical Trial. JAMA 2016; 315: 1266.
157. Mandel JS, Church TR, Bond JH, Ederer F, Geisser MS, Mongin SJ et al. The effect of fecal occult-blood screening on the incidence of colorectal cancer. New England Journal of Medicine 2000; 343(22):1603-1607.
158. De Gramont A, Andre T, Housset M, Nordlinger B, Rougier P. Colorectal cancer in questions. Fondation ARCAD 2015; 3rd Ed: 8-10
159. Faivre J, Lepagea C, Viguier, G. Colorectal cancer: from diagnosis to screening Clinical and Biological Gastroenterology 2009; 33, 660-671
160. Launoy G. Advances in colorectal cancer screening related to the use of new immunological tests for blood in stool. Pathologie Biologie 2008; 488-492.
161. Kim GH, Liang PS, Bang SJ, Hwang JH. Gastric cancer screening and surveillance in the United States: is it necessary? Gastrointest Endosc. 2016; 84: 18-28.
162. Hamashima C. Systematic review G. Guideline development group for gastric cancer screening G. Updated version of the Japanese guidelines for gastric cancer screening. Jpn J Clin Oncol. 2018; 48: 673-83.
163. Greenhalf W, Grocock C, Harcus M, Neoptolemos J. Screening families at high risk for pancreatic cancer. Pancreatology. 2009; 9 (3): 215-222. doi: 10.1159 / 000210262.
164. Shin EJ, Canto MI. Pancreatic cancer screening. Gastroenterol Clin North Am. 2012; 41 (1): 143-157. doi: 10.1016 / j.gtc.2011.12.001.
165. Basturk, O., Hong, S. M., Wood, L. D., Adsay, N. V., Albores-Saavedra, J., Biankin, A. V.,Baltimore Consensus, M. (2015). A Revised Classification System and Recommendations From the Baltimore Consensus Meeting for Neoplastic Precursor Lesions in the Pancreas. Am J Surg

Pathol, 39(12), 1730-1741. doi:10.1097/PAS. 533.
166. European Study Group on Cystic Tumours of the, P. (2018). European evidence-based guidelines on pancreatic cystic neoplasms. Gut, 67(5), 789-804. doi:10.1136/gutjnl-2018-316027.
167. Serife Koc, Melek Nihal Esin and Aysun Ardic.Colorectal Cancer Prevention and Risk CounselingSubmitted: October 5th 2015Reviewed: March 18th 2016Published: September 7th 2016 DOI: 10.5772/63206
168. Cindy Neuzillet Hopitaux Universitaires Paris Nord Val de Seine (HUPNVS), Universite Paris 7 - Hopital Beaujon, Denis Diderot, INSERM UMR1149 and service d'oncologie digestive, 100 boulevard du General Leclerc, 92110 Clichy La Garenne, France. 10.1684/hpg.2017.1428 page. 249-58.
169. Sante maghreb.com. Guide de sante en ALGERIE, Les registres du cancer en Afrique)
170. National Network of Cancer Registries. Ministere de la sante et de la reforme hospitaliere, Alger 2016
171. Hammouda D, Aoun MD, Bouzerar K, Namaoui M, Rezzik I, et al. Registre des tumeurs d'Alger annee 2006.
172. International Classification of Diseases for Oncology, Third Edition, eds. Fritz A, Percy C, Jack A, et al. Geneva, World Health Organization, 2000.
173. Morten JE. CanReg 5 Manual. IARC 2008-2013. International Agency for Research on Cancer. 2014; World health organization.
174. J. Ferlay, C. Burkhard, S. Whelan, D.M. Parkin, Check And Conversion Programs For Cancer Registries. Iarc//Iacr Tools for Cancer Registries, IARC Technical Report No. 42 Lyon, 2005.
175. Guidelines on confidentiality for population-based cancer registries. Internal Report No. 2004 / 03, IARC Lyon 2004 http://www.iacr.com.fr/confidentiality2004. pdf.
176. Hyem Khiari, Rym Mallekh, Mohamed Hsairi ,Service d'Epidemiologie, Institut Salah Azaiz-Tunis.Strategies of the Maghreb countries in the fight against cancer .LA TUNISIE MEDICALE - 2021 ; Vol 99 (n°01).
177. Ministere de la Sante .Plan pour la lutte contre le cancer 2015-2019 [Online]. Tunis, Ministry of Health; 2015 [cited 25 September 2020]. Available from URL:https://www.iccp-portal.org/system/files/plans/Plan_ pour_la_lutte_contre_le_cancer_2015-2019_Tunisie.pdf.
178. Ministere de la Sante .Plan national de prévention et de contrôle du cancer 20102019: Axes strategiques et mesures [Online]. Rabat, Ministere de la sante; 2009 [cited 2020 Sep 25]. Available from URL: http://www.contrelecancer.ma/site media/uploaded-files/PNPCC_-_Axes_strategiques_et_mesures_2010-2019.pdf
179. M .Hamdi Cherif, et Col, Données d'incidence du reseau National des Registres du Cancer, Algerie ,2015 ; Revue El hakim numero hors série, Vol II, Avril 2018.
180. Descriptive epidemiology of cancers in the Maghreb (Algeria, Morocco, Tunisia) M Hamdi Cherif, C Nejjari, M BenAbdallah, W Ben Ayoub, H Sancho-Garnier,Maghreb Review. Vol. 34, 2010.
181. Cancer in the Maghreb and the Middle East at the Heart of the Epidemiological Transition Mokhtar Hamdi Cherif Edition: Editions universitaires europeennes (28-06-2017), June 2017 ISBN: ISBN-13: 978-3-33087817-4.
182. Surveillance epidemiologique des cancers : Resultats preliminaires nationaux D. Hammouda* ; L. Boutekdjiret Coordinatrice du reseau centre des registres des cancers, INSP Alger. Algerian Journal of Health Sciences volume 2. 2020
183. Global Burden of Disease Cancer Collaboration, Fitzmaurice C, Allen C, et al. Global, regional, and national cancer incidence, mortality, years of life lost, years lived with disability, and disability-adjusted life years for 32 cancer groups, 1990 to 2015: a systematic analysis for the study of the global burden of disease. JAMA Oncol 2017; 3: 524.

184. Sheh A, Ge Z, Parry NM, et al. 17beta-estradiol and tamoxifen prevent gastric cancer by modulating leukocyte recruitment and oncogenic pathways in Helicobacter pylori-infected INS-GAS male mice. Cancer Prev Res (Phila) 2011;4:1426-35.

185. Minicozzi P, Cassetti T, Vener C, Sant M. Analysis of incidence, mortality and survival for pancreatic and biliary tract cancers across Europe, with assessment of influence of revised European agestandardisation on estimates. Cancer Epidemiol. August 2018;55:52-60

186. Sharma A, Sharma KL, Gupta A, Yadav A, Kumar A. Gallbladder cancer epidemiology, pathogenesis and molecular genetic, Recent update. World J Gastroenterol. June 2017;23(22):3978-98.

187. Bray F, Colombet M, Mery L, Pineros M, Znaor A, Zanetti R and Ferlay J, editors (2017). Cancer Incidence in Five Continents, Vol.XI (electronic version). Lyon: International Agency for Research on Cancer. Available from URL: http://ci5.iarc.fr

188. Ezzati M, Henley SJ, Lopez AD, Thun MJ. Role of smoking in global and regional cancer epidemiology: current trends and data needs. Int J Cancer. 2005; 116 (6): 963-971. doi: 10.1002 / ijc.21100.

189. Willett WC. Diet and cancer. Oncologist. 2000; 5 (5): 393-404. doi: 10.1634 / theoncologue.5-5-393.

190. Avgerinos DV, Bjornsson J. malignant neoplasms: discordance between clinical diagnoses and autopsy findings in 3118 case. APMIS. 2001; 109 (11): 774-780. doi: 10.1034 / j.1600-0463.2001.d01-145.x.

191. Mathers CD, Fat DM, Inoue M, Rao C, Lopez AD. Counting the dead and what they died of: an assessment of the global status of cause-of-death data. World Health Organization Bull. 2005; 83 (3): 171-177.

192. Ferlay J, Steliarova-Foucher E, Lortet-Tieulent J, Rosso S, Coebergh JW, Comber H, Forman D. et al. Cancer incidence and mortality patterns in Europe: estimates for 40 countries in 2012. Eur J Cancer. 2013; 49 (6): 1374-1403. doi: 10.1016 / j.ejca.2012.12.027.

193. Forner A, Reig M, Bruix J. Hepatocellular carcinoma. Lancet.March 2018; 391(10127):1301-14.

194. Bertuccio P, Turati F, Carioli G, Rodriguez T, La Vecchia C, Malvezzi M, et al.Global trends and predictions in hepatocellular carcinoma mortality. J Hepatol. August 2017;67(2):3029.

195. Dong J, Thrift AP. Alcohol, smoking and risk of oesophago-gastric cancer. Best Pract Res Clin Gastroenterol. 2017; 31(5):509-17.

196. Walker RC, Underwood TJ. Oesophageal cancer. Surgery-Oxford International Edition. 2017;35(11): 627-34

197. Reynolds I, Healy P, Mcnamara DA. Malignant tumours of the small intestine. Surgeon. Oct 2014;12(5):263-70.

198. Balakrishnan M, George R, Sharma A, Graham DY. Changing trends in stomach cancer throughout the world. Curr Gastroenterol Rep. 2017;19:36.

ANNEX I
Description of the East & South East region and population

Description of the East & South-East region:

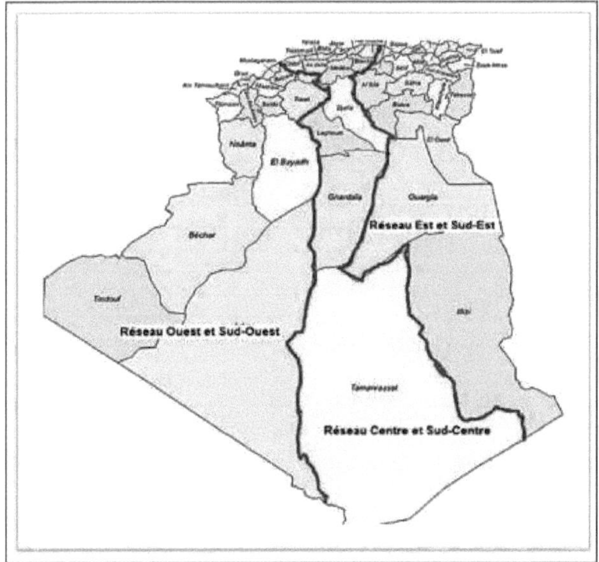

The East and South East network comprises 20 wilayas and geographically it is divided into three main reliefs: the Tell, the Highlands and the Sahara:

Geography of the network :

The eastern Tell extends from Bejaia to El Taraf. It is dominated by the mountains of Petite Kabylie and is characterised by a very mountainous appearance, leaving very little room for small coastal plains (Bejaia, Jijel, Skikda, Annaba) or inner basins squeezed behind steep defiles (Rummel, El-Kebir, Seybouse). From the nuclei of ancient massifs, straightened and deeply dissected by erosion, fall the powerful limestone "sierras" of the Bibans and the discontinuous limestone chain of the Babors, which carry the highest peaks to more than 2,000 m. This region, the most densely mountainous of all Algeria, is also the most humid. Water of 1 to 2 m falls annually on these djebels, often in the form of snow. The highest peaks are covered with cedar forests, but the wet, siliceous slopes of the Collo and Edough peninsulas are covered with thick, scrubby undergrowth of oak forests. It is here, par excellence, the Algeria of the great djebels, humid and wooded.

The High Plains of the Interior lie between the Tell and the Presaharan mountains, which separate them from the desert. They are 200 km wide and rise from 1,000 m to 1,200 m. The conditions of the relief change at the same time as those of the climate. Behind the shelter of the Tellian Atlas, precipitation decreases quite significantly (less than 500 mm, but most often less than 400 mm). It becomes increasingly irregular and low towards the south. The altitude and continental nature of the region accentuate the temperature contrasts between day and night (daily amplitude much higher than on the coast), but also between summer and winter (very high summer temperatures with maximums above 40°C; cold winters with many days of frost). The steppe is the usual vegetation of the high plains, a low formation composed of low plants that do not cover the ground well and are adapted to the drought (mugwort, esparto grass, etc.). The Presaharan mountains, especially the higher ones, receive some additional rainfall. They also have, above the steppe or scrubby lower slopes, open forests of holm oak and Aleppo pine, and even some cedar forests on certain summits (Aures).

Demographics :

Population estimates by wilaya of the East and South-East Algerian network (2017).

Register of the Wilaya of :	Population covered		
	Female	Male	Both sexes
Setif	881438	883840	1 765278
Constantine	566006	563477	1 129 483
Bejaia	542642	519956	1 062 598
Batna	683295	669342	1 352637
Annaba	359223	358358	717 581
Jijel	380832	374597	755 429
Ouargla	351744	340384	692128
Biskra	452888	440967	893 855
Khenchela	237181	231618	468 799
Oum El Bouaghi	383812	375323	759135
Tebessa	395588	390874	786 462
Skikda	543129	534508	1 077637
Guelma	288733	285540	574273
Msila	621928	596656	1218584
Illizi	37905	32279	70184
BBA	383785	367084	750869
El Taref	245582	245956	491538
El Oued	413656	397517	811173
Souk Ahras	266491	266618	533109
Mila	462255	453981	916236
East and South-East Region	8498113	8328875	16826988

Health coverage :

The national health system, which is the set of activities and means intended to ensure the protection and promotion of the population's health, is organised in such a way as to be able to take charge of the population's health needs in a global, coherent and unified manner within the framework of **the health map**. In principle, it is designed according to its objectives, which are the improvement of the health of the population, equity and the capacity to meet the legitimate expectations of the population.

North East Region: which includes the 09 wilayas of : Annaba, Bejaia, Constantine, El Taraf, Guelma, Jijel, Skikda, Souk-Ahras, Mila.

Region	Superfine	Population 2014	Hospitals N. of beds	Polyclinic	Treatment room	Maternity	CAC
North East 9 wilayas	25,945 km^2 1,2%	05.747.816 15,8 %	42 04CHU* 37 EPH 11 EHS 11843 beds 2 beds/lOOOh	260 l/22106h.	1026 l/5602h	50 (401 beds)	03

Eastern Highlands region: which includes the 06 wilayas of : Batna, Bordj Bou Arreridj, Oum El Bouaghi, Khenchela, Setif, Tebessa.

Region	Area	Population 2014	Hospitals	Polyclinic	Treatment room	Maternity	CAC
Highlands East 6 wilayas 6	54,487 km^2 2,3%	5.556.075 15,2 %	50 02 UNIVERSITY HOSPITAL 36 EPH 12 EHS 9715 beds l,7lits/1000h	248 1/22403H.	1013 1/5484K	83 (697 beds)	02

South East Region: which includes the 05 wilayas of : El Oued, Biskra, Ouargla, Illizi, Tamanrasset **(but for the network the wilaya of Tamanrasset is part of the central network)**.

Region	Area	Population 2014	Hospitals	Polyclinic	Treatment room	Integrated Maternity	CAC
South East 05 wilayas	1.130.063 Km^2 47,4%	2.346.811 6,4 %	22 16EPH+06 EHS 3464 beds 1.3 beds/lOOOh	110 1/21334K.	443 l/5295h	38 227 beds	01

ANNEX II

Cancer notification form

The ministerial order to institutionalise population registers

National Cancer Plan 2015 - 2019

REGISTRE DU CANCER DE SETIF, ALGERIE

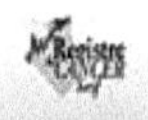

Directeur : Pr M. Hamdi-chérif,
Service d'Epidémiologie et de Médecine Préventive,
CHU de Sétif, Sétif, Algérie.
Tél/Fax: +213 36 61 61 76

En collaboration avec le Centre International de Recherche sur le Cancer, Lyon, France.

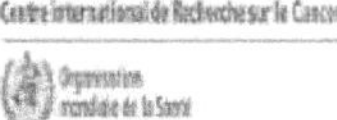

1. NUMERO MATRICULE	(laisser en blanc)	/_/_/_/_/_/_/
2. SOURCE D'INFORMATION		
01 CHU de Sétif	10 Certificat de décès	
02 EPSP, EPH Wilaya	11 Fichier National	
03 Labo. Anapath, CHU.	12 CPMC Alger	
04 Oncologie CLCC	13 Associations	
05 Radiothérapie CLCC	14 Autres CHU	
06 Chirurgie CLCC	15 Labo. Anapath, CLCC	
07 CLCC proche	16 Hématologie CLCC	
08 Labo. Anapath privé	17 Autre (préciser)	
09 Clinique privée		/_/_/
3. NUMERO DE SOURCE..............		/_/_/_/_/_/_/_/
4. NOM..............		
5. PRENOM..............		
6. SEXE (1=masculin, 2=féminin, 3=autre, 9=inconnu)		/_/
7. PROFESSION..............		/_/_/_/
8. DATE DE NAISSANCE (jour-mois-année)..............		/_/_/_/_/_/_/
9. AGE..............		/_/_/
10. ADRESSE..............		
11. DAIRA..............COMMUNE..............		/_/_/_/_/
12. NUMERO DE TÉLÉPHONE..............		/_/_/_/_/_/_/_/_/_/_/
13. DATE DE DIAGNOSTIC (jour/mois/année)..............		/_/_/_/_/_/_/
14. LOCALISATION..............		/_/_/_/_/
15. MORPHOLOGIE..............		/_/_/_/_/_/
16. Classification TNM..............		T/__/__/N/__/__/M/__/__/
16. BASE DE DIAGNOSTIC		Grade/_____/_____/
00 Certificat de décès uniquement	01 Clinique	
02 Investigation clinique (radiologie, endoscopies...)		
03 Chirurgie/Autopsie Sans pathologie	04 Biochimique/ Immunologie.	
05 Cytologie/Hématologie	06 Pathologie de métastase	
07 Pathologie de tumeur primitive	08 Autopsie avec pathologie	/_/_/
09 Inconnu	10 Autre (préciser)	
17. SUIVI (1=vivant, 2=mort, 9=inconnu)..............		/_/
18. DATE DE SUIVI (jour-mois-année)..............		/_/_/_/_/_/_/
19. CAUSE DE DECES..............		/_/_/_/_/
20. ENQUETEUR..............		/_/_/

(Codage central, laisser ces cases en blanc)

REPUBLIQUE ALGERIENNE DEMOCRATIQUE ET POPULAIRE
MINISTERE DE LA SANTE LA POPULATION ET DE LA REFORME HOSPITALIERE

17 MARS 2014

ARRETE N° 95 DU 17 MARS 2014 PORTANT CREATION, FONCTIONNEMENT ET ORGANISATION DU REGISTRE DU CANCER DE POPULATION

Le secrétaire général,

- Vu la loi n° 85-05 du 26 djoumada El Aoula 1405 correspondant au 16 février 1985, modifiée et complétée, relative à la protection et à la promotion de la santé,
- Vu le décret exécutif n°93-153 du 08 Moharam 1414 correspondant au 28 juin 1993 portant création du Bulletin Officiel du Ministère de la Santé et de la Population,
- Vu la loi n° 12-07 du 28 Rabie El Aouel 1433 correspondant au 21 février 2012 relative à la wilaya ;
- Vu le décret présidentiel n°13-312 du 5 Dhou El Kaâda 1434 correspondant au 11 septembre 2013 portant nomination des membres du Gouvernement;
- Vu le décret exécutif n°11-379 du 25 dhou elhidja 1432 correspondant au 21 novembre 2011 fixant les attributions du Ministre de la Santé, de la Population et de la Réforme Hospitalière,
- Vu le décret exécutif n°11-380 du 25 dhou elhidja 1432 correspondant au 21 novembre 2011 portant organisation de l'administration centrale du Ministère de la Santé, de la Population et de la Réforme Hospitalière
- Vu l'arrêté n° 08 du 14 janvier 2013 portant création du collège national d'experts et des comités d'experts en santé.

ARRETE

ARTICLE 1. Il est crée au niveau de chaque wilaya, un registre du cancer de population dénommé, ci-après, le « Registre ».

ARTICLE 2. Le Registre est chargé de procéder à la collecte, au stockage et à l'interprétation des données relatives aux malades atteints de cancer dans un territoire donné.

ARTICLE 3 : Le Registre est positionné au niveau du Service d'Epidémiologie et de Médecine Préventive des CHU et des EPH chef-lieu des wilayas non dotées de CHU à l'exception de la wilaya d'Alger ou il est positionné au niveau de l'INSP.

ARTICLE 4 : Les missions du Registre sont de :

- assurer l'enregistrement exhaustif et prospectif de tous les cancers de la wilaya dans sa limite géographique,
- fournir des données fiables et standardisées des cancers de la wilaya,
- constituer une banque de données utiles pour les décideurs, les prestataires et les chercheurs,
- susciter et conduire des études épidémiologiques visant à vérifier certaines hypothèses étiologiques,
- étudier la tendance de l'incidence de la mortalité et de la survie,
- estimer les besoins et prévisions en soins et les coûts financiers

ARTICLE 5 : Le Registre est placé sous la responsabilité du chef de service d'épidémiologie et de médecine préventive des établissements ou il est positionné.

ARTICLE 6 : Le Directeur de la Santé et de la Population de wilaya est tenu à ce que les établissements dont relève le Registre soient dotés en moyens humains et matériels pour son bon fonctionnement.

ARTICLE 7: Le fonctionnement du registre nécessite les moyens humains et matériels suivants :

- au minimum de (2) deux médecins et (2) deux techniciens,
- un microordinateur,
- le logiciel standardisé spécifique recommandé par l'OMS,
- un véhicule chaque fois que de besoin pour le recueil actif des données,
- des moyens de communication et de reprographie.

ARTICLE 8: Les responsables des services chargés de l'exploration, du diagnostic, du traitement et du suivi de la maladie cancéreuse du secteur public, parapublique et privé sont tenus de faciliter l'accès à l'information aux personnels chargés du Registre

ARTICLE 9 : Le fonctionnement du Registre demande une rigueur éthique, les données nominatives qui relèvent de la maladie sont répertoriés dans un fichier spécial et confidentiel.

ARTICLE 10: Les Registres sont organisés en un réseau national dénommé « Réseau National des Registres du Cancer de Population ».

ARTICLE 11 : La coordination du Réseau National des Registres du Cancer de Population est placée auprès de la Direction Générale de la Prévention et de la Promotion de la Santé chargée de consolider les données de la situation du cancer à l'échelle nationale.

ARTICLE 12 : Le responsable du Registre est tenu de transmettre à la Direction Générale de la Prévention et de la Promotion de la Santé :

- un rapport trimestriel sur les données de la situation du registre du cancer de la wilaya
- un rapport annuel des données d'incidence du cancer

ARTICLE 13 : Le présent arrêté sera publié au Bulletin Officiel du Ministère de la Santé et de la Population.

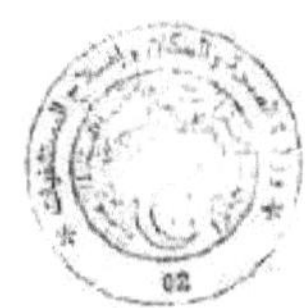

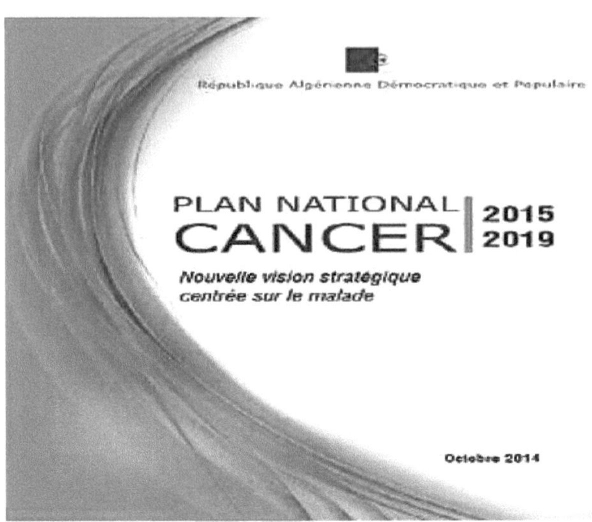
République Algérienne Démocratique et Populaire
PLAN NATIONAL CANCER
2015
2019
Nouvelle vision stratégique
centrée sur le malade
Octobre 2014

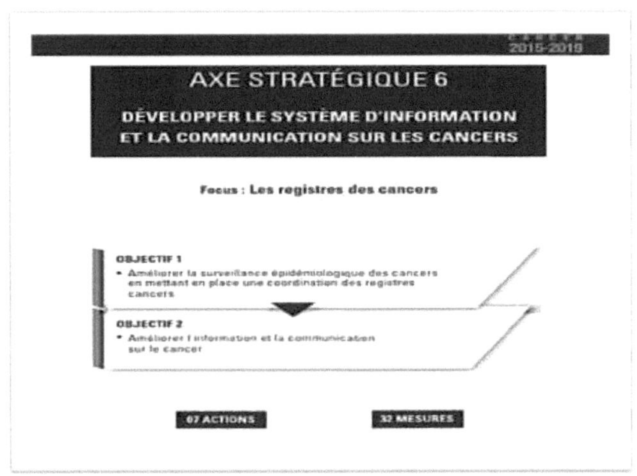
2015-2019
AXE STRATÉGIQUE 6
DÉVELOPPER LE SYSTÈME D'INFORMATION
ET LA COMMUNICATION SUR LES CANCERS
Focus : Les registres des cancers
OBJECTIF 1
• Améliorer la surveillance épidémiologique des cancers en mettant en place une coordination des registres cancers
OBJECTIF 2
• Améliorer l'information et la communication sur le cancer
07 ACTIONS
32 MESURES

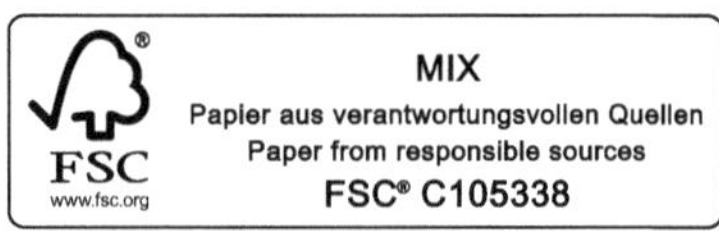

Printed by Books on Demand GmbH, Norderstedt / Germany